HEALTH CARE IN INDIAN POLICE FORCES
An Analysis of Problems and Perspectives

HEALTH CARE IN INDIAN POLICE FORCES

An Analysis of Problems and Perspectives

G.C. SATPATHY, M.D. (Medicine)

Foreword by

D.R. KARTHIKEYAN, IPS
Additional Director General, CRPF

GYAN

GYAN PUBLISHING HOUSE

NEW DELHI-110002

Health Care in Indian Police Forces
An Analysis of Problems and Perspectives
(Police, Public Administration , Medicine Health)

ISBN: 81-212-0467-4
Library of Congress Card No. 93-900322

Published in 1994 by
Gyan Publishing House
5 Ansari Road
New Delhi 110 002

Laser typesetting at Jeetu Graphics, Delhi- 110 094, and printed at Goyal Offset Works, Delhi-110 022

FOREWORD

Dr. G.C. Satpathy, M.D. (Medicine), in the CRPF Group Centre Hospital at Neemuch has attempted an analysis of the problems and perspectives of health care in the premier para military force-CRPF.

In the very first chapter, the author has in very general terms traced the history of Medicine and Police from varied times and their subsequent growth through ancient, medieval and modern times. The author also highlights the neglect in Police health care due to scepticism prevailing amongst policy makers. However, it is a moot point whether the negligence in Police health care is due to criticism among policy makers or due to lack of planning or lack of resources.

A cursory reading of this book gives one impression that the title ought to have been more appropriately Health Care in CRPF rather than Health Care in Indian Police Forces. I find some of the conclusions drawn by the author in the field of general policing is mainly based on his experiences in the CRPF.

The author refers to actions of Police men against their will and conscience and being compelled to do so by the senior administrators. This obviously is based on some of his odd personal experiences in certain insurgency infected areas. Perhaps, he may not be right in drawing a general conclusion for the Police Forces as a whole from such stray experiences.

He has, however, highlighted factors which lead to certain diseases among policemen, especially stress factors. He has also underlined the role of doctors in keeping the force healthy through not only preventive and curative treatments but also health education. The author has also laid importance on the need for higher studies among Medical Officers in CPOs. There is also the need for the Medical Officers to update their knowledge of advances in medical research through Medical journals and by participation in seminars and workshops.

Using his experience in the CRPF Dr. Satpathy has covered functions of various field and base medical formations in this prestigious Force. Procurement of hospital stores, general stores, medical stores and diets for patients are all dealt with in detail. The need and importance of annual health checks, special problems of women members of the force and aid to civilians during natural calamities also find mention in the book.

In Chapter 10, he refers to the impact of various diseases on police duties. According to Dr. Satpathy, Malaria causes more damage to the force personnel than enemy action. He could have given statistics to show the adverse effect of Malaria vis-a-vis casualties in action which could have given an impetus to the disease eradication programmes. The Author has appealed for specialised hospital management, arranging visits of specialists to Police hospitals and exchange programmes with reputed hospitals for training police doctors. He has also rightly called for encouraging alternate medical systems like Unani, Ayurveda and Homoeopathy.

He feels that an integrated command and control of Hospitals of various CPOs would serve para-military medical services better by removing disparity in service conditions and ensuring uniformity in service conditions of hospital staff. He has also appealed for continuous modernisation, better planning in group health insurance schemes and utilisation of retired but active police officers gainfully.

On the whole, I am quite impressed by the study made by the author and the efforts put in by him to highlight the need for proper health care in Police Forces. I am sure this work will initiate more studies in depth on this very important subject.

Hyderabad

D.R. KARTHIKEYAN, IPS
Additional Director General
Central Reserve Police Force
Southern Sector

PREFACE

Police has been the executive arm of the administration for centuries. The post-independent decades have seen the formation and growth of police forces with cancerous rapidity almost parallel to the lawlessness and terrorism. More and more specialised, equipped, sophisticated wings are being added to the spectrum of armed and unarmed police forces every year. The special task forces like National Security Guards (NSG), Rapid Action Force (RAF) in CRPF, rise of women battalions, etc. are the latest additions to the fighting police troops. Airport Security Force and India Reserve Battalions are on the cards. The coming years may see many such experiments. The police forces are constantly fighting an "Undeclared War" in our own streets. They are the vigilant sentries in our frontiers facing all hardships in life, separated from kith and kin. For the dynamic nature of duties, the police forces are to be kept physically fit, mentally happy and alert and morally sound. The greater police family spreads from the home guards to civil police, plain cloth policemen, state armed forces to the Central Para-military forces with their specialised wings. The health care of this vast police family has been a challenge to the planners of police policies and leaders at the helm of affairs.

The police forces have to constantly maintain a high health profile to face the challenge of lawlessness and terrorism.

A devoted group of medical and para-medical personnels are engaged day and night to maintain the health care service in the police forces like behind-the-scene green room boys. They provide an efficient clinical and public health service ensuring the best of health and well being of troops, preserve agility and fitness in them. The medical science as well as the police technics are advancing so rapidly with time, unless the wing of medical service in police forces keep on advancing at right pace, the service will lag behind. Its advancement needs thorough research on every aspect of the service. Hence, it is an open invitation to the thinkers of police and medical sciences of the present world to pay due attention to the police health care services.

Unfortunately, the thinkers of modern day police are yet to devote their time on the vital issue of police health which concerns the vast police population and their families. The men in uniform have their own occupational health problems and on the other hand. the diseases have their impact over the police duty. Health of women troops, sports persons, recruits, etc. have their own peculiarities. Hence, the task as a whole is enormous.

My two decades long association with the police force has made me to go through the available police literatures in many units, group headquarters, academies, training centres, etc. Our cupboards are full of police principles, philosophies, morals, training methods, experience and memoirs of veteran police officers. They speak of the failures and achievements of police forces in civil and frontier operations. But it was painful for me to find that the coverage of the police health care system has been grossly inadequate. Such a situation has compelled me to start a trend from a scratch. No worth referable literature is available on the subject. Hence, the present writing is largely based on my experiences, gathered from work and study made in own force and sister organisations. Multiple aspects of the system have been analysed for its pros and cons; criticised frankly and bitterly at times; praised the worthy ones with no exaggerations and suggestions have been forwarded without waiting for anybody to accept; gone deep to probe the colics felt under the khaki uniform and frost bites under the heavy snow boots. This is the content of the book.

But all said and done, the medical service still occupies a back seat in police heirarchy. Ad-hocism still prevails. "Borrowed" medical system still persists. How long can the police forces march with the hang-over of a Grade II Army ? It is high time that the planners of police forces do away with their symptomatic remedy and loose sheet planning. Their approach needs to be more realistic and practical. With massive upsurge of militancy in the country, the future police forces need to be fit and healthy enough to face the challenge, otherwise, the future peace keepers would curse them and the country will be in total chaos. We can never be the mute witness to the heavy police casualties as the police forces are constantly fighting an undeclared war.

I have been working shoulder to shoulder with the khaki-clad citizens of CRPF for last two decades. The Police Force environment has visible impact on my life-style, so also my writings. Hence, the narrations of health care in this book is grossly CPO oriented and CRPF based. I am grateful to my numerous friends, doctors colleagues associates, patients, trainees of my own force and sister forces including some state police establishments, who have largely contributed to improve my information on the working of Health Care Systems. This is no exaggeration to say that this work would not have been possible without their unconditional and liberal support. If this work benefits the organisations or helps in improvement of the medical organisations it would be rightly considered a success.

I am vastly indebted and grateful to honourable Shri D.R. Karthikeyan, IPS Addl. D.G. CRPF and Chief of SIT Rajiv Gandhi Assassination Case, one of the most distinguished police officer in the country of present time, having spared his time to go through the draft, and write the foreword for the book. Lastly, as a physician's life is rarely congenial for concentrating on writing work such an atmosphere has been made possible by my wife who deserves thanks.

G.C. SATPATHY

CONTENTS

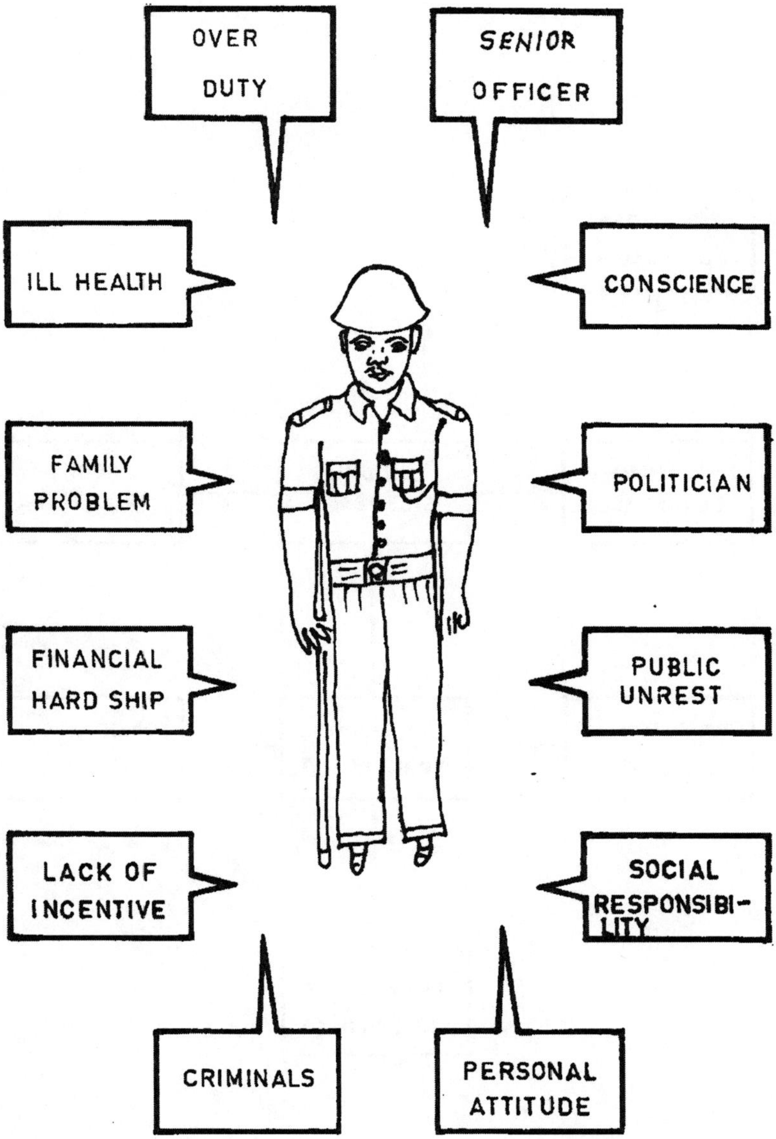
OVER DUTY
SENIOR OFFICER
ILL HEALTH
CONSCIENCE
FAMILY PROBLEM
POLITICIAN
FINANCIAL HARD SHIP
PUBLIC UNREST
LACK OF INCENTIVE
SOCIAL RESPONSIBI-LITY
CRIMINALS
PERSONAL ATTITUDE

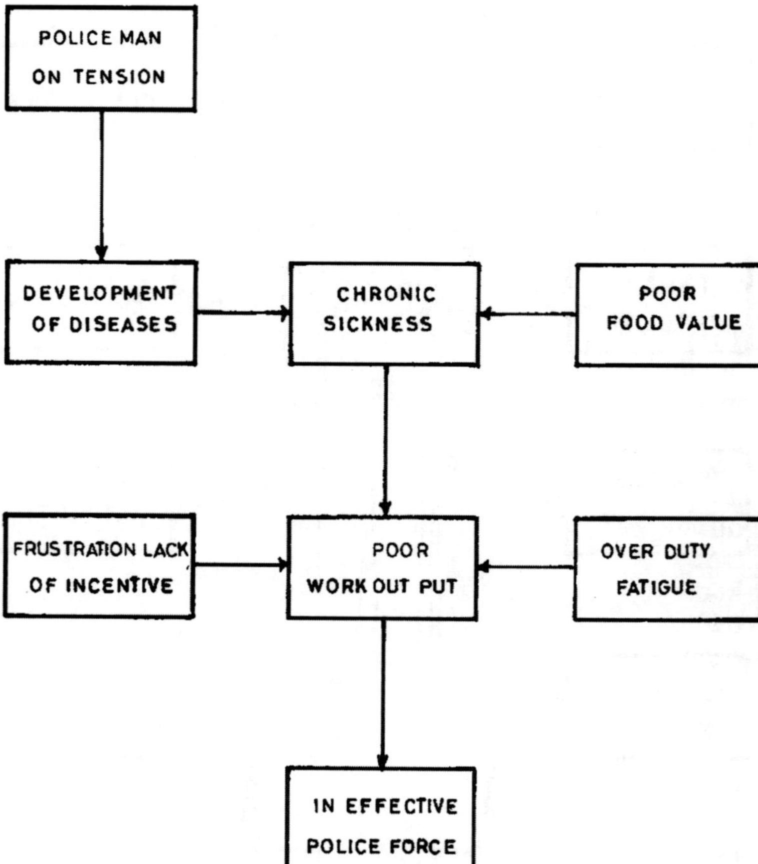
POLICE MAN ON TENSION
DEVELOPMENT OF DISEASES
CHRONIC SICKNESS
POOR FOOD VALUE
FRUSTRATION LACK OF INCENTIVE
POOR WORK OUT PUT
OVER DUTY FATIGUE
IN EFFECTIVE POLICE FORCE

1

March of Medicine and Police (Some Foot Prints, Some Landmarks)

The origin of concepts of health and police is deeply embedded in antiquity, historical antecedents and evolutionary changes in Indian Society. Medicine is the application of scientific knowledge and technical knowhow for the prevention and amelioration of human damage and suffering. Whereas police is a system of regulation, preservation of order and enforcement of law of the State. Medicine and police are perceived by many of their practitioners to be two distinct doctrines of knowledge and scientific application. The alliance between the two is not easily digested. It is not only mutual mistrust, but a poor comprehension of the striking resemblance between their professional philosophies. A physician is trained to diagnose a physiological abnormality and curing of the illness, whereas a police officer discovers the social malady and plans for remedying the same. Because of the prevailing scepticism which clouds the vision of police policy makers as well as the medical professionals, there is unpardonable negligence in the field of police health care which is of utmost significance in contemporary society. The parallels of the two professions intersect at many points like camp sanitation, health education, Forensic Medicine, immunisation, personal hygiene, public health measures, sports medicine, recruitment to armed forces, invalidation, philanthropic service and a host of other fields. This field of vital human concern lacks serious research and hence the problems faced by the health care machinery in police forces remain unanswered.

The history of medicine is long enough to cover the entire story of civilization. The earliest concepts are described in *Atharva Veda*. King Dhanwantari learnt *Ayurveda* (Science of Life) from Brahma. The classic ancient Indian literatures like *Charaka Samhita* and *Susruta Samhita* are the earliest medical records available to the world of medicine and surgery, treated superior to Greek Medical antics, which later influenced the western world. Both these works are comprehensive and illustrate the three universal forces regulating human systems, such as *Kapha* (Phlegm), *Pitta* (Bile) and *Vayu* (Air). The derangement of any or more than one of these forces lead to illness and the treatments are also aimed at correcting the basic disorders. Other Hindu writings spell about diagnostic procedures and prognostic assessment at length. The therapeutics are basically of dietetic and medicinal in nature. Most treatments consisted of procedures such as emetics, enema, purgatives and sneezing procedures. The Indian *materia medica* includes vegetable drugs, drugs prepared from various animal products like milk of different animals, *Kasturi*, minerals like gold, carbon, arsenic, lead, copper, sulphur, etc. Scientist Charaka has described utility of 500 plants and Susruta of 760 in the preparation of herbo-mineral medicines. Modern surgery owes to the contribution of Susruta who recommended 20 sharp and 101 blunt instruments. Surgery of urinary stones, anal fistulla and plastic surgery were practiced in India by Hindu surgeons much before the Greeks.

The principle of hygiene and sanitation were followed in India as part of their social customs and religious observance, derived from ayurvedic literatures. The system teaches complete health care procedures covering all stages, aspects and parts of life and body. The teachings attracted numerous disciples from abroad where they carried the science and propagated, giving India the status of sole health educator in the then world. Unfortunately, in India itself, the science was fading away due to lack of patronisation and influence of western medicine till it was revived in subsequent centuries.

During Muslim rule, *Yunani* system of medicine came to India from Greece and was confined to Muslim population. The founders of this system were from Persia, Arabia, Italy and Greece. They include Hippocrates, who is also worshiped as the Father of Modern Medicine. The scientific research and professional development over the ancient systems of medicine lead to the new world of "Modern Medicine", initially called European Medicine. The entry of the newly developed health care science to India was possible through the Dutch, French and Spanish travellers and missionaries prior to 5th Century. i.e., much before East India Company was established. The 17th Century saw the decline of Mughal Empire and the British Crown gaining control over Indian sub-continent. The British Rule over India for centuries introduced several significant changes including creation of class of professionals in medical science.

The civilised people of Indus Valley had knowledge of planned city life and public health facilities five thousand years ago. Their household had bathroom, latrine, carefully built wells and drainage system, signifying great emphasis on preventive aspects of diseases, and mature attitude to health problems. The famous rock edicts of Emperor Ashoka also describes principles of social medicine in the line of Buddhist thought and teachings. Even in the epic *Mahabharata*, the principles of hygiene were enforced by Senapati Karna and hence he is worshipped as the first Military Hygienist known to the world.

During the subsequent centuries, series of socio-political and economic changes in the country greatly influenced the overall social and health culture. The history of health services in India provides an account of all such forces. Other systems as *Siddha* (practiced by *Sadhus*) and Homeopathy, a German system of medicine were also in practice in India. Inspite of presence of several systems of medicine, indigenous or otherwise, the allopathy or modern medicine had the worldwide acceptance and dominated the Indian scene, with full patronisation from British rulers because of its scientific character and rational theories and formulations. The British rulers subjected every facts of life, including medical and public health services to their commercial, political and administrative interests which was a fatal blow to Indian system of medicine. In fact, the Indian system of medicine could not compete the highly advanced western system which came as total replacement to the former. The western medicine not only brought radical cure and comfort to the suffering mass, it captured the imagination of the educated population of India. In absence of proper training facilities, the practice of modern medicine suffered from infiltration by quacks leading to erosion of scientific values.

The benefits of modern allopathic medicine were available to the native Indian population much later, where as medical services were established to support the British Army and British civilian personnel living in India, in the later half of 18th century. The personnel of Indian medical service of British days were called upon to initiate a new health service system for common mass. The medical education facility was available to very priviledged upper class of society and higher education in Britain was again for the "Select of the Select". Acquiring membership or fellowship in various Royal Colleges used to be the pinnacle of achievement in their respective fields. To the Indian physicians, the medical diploma ensured power, prestige, status and money. They (somebody described them as the "Brown Englishmen") held the key positions and had meteoric rise after the British left India for good. In the post independent India, the medical service and medical education, training of para-medical staff and development of other health infra-structures like manufacture of essential drugs have been thoroughly revolutionised, modernised and expanded. The priority of health of rural mass was emphasised in Five Year Plans and mass campaign against major health hazards like small pox, malaria, tuberculosis and family planning achieved demographic objectives with reasonable marginal failures.

Inspite of several remedial measures, the country's health care facilities are still to reach the remotest corners and are still beyond affordable scope of poorest of the poor. About 80 per cent products of medical colleges prefer to serve the 20 per cent population of city dwellers. Unfortunately, the imbalance is in rise. When the villages lack the basic health facilities, the cities and megacities go for most modern electro-medical technologies and computer application for diagnostic and therapeutic purposes. Some limited centres in private and public sectors have CAT Scan, Magnetic Resonance Imaging (MRI), and conduct EEG, EMG, Angiography, Mammography, Lithotripsy, cardiac and brain surgery, etc. The dynamic health experts take initiatives to offer the best medical facilities to the public. It is upto the common man to avail it. With the media playing role of health guide, the health consciousness has increased *vis-a-vis* with health needs. The accessibility, affordability and the quality of health care service are the three crucial factors in the health care system in the country. There is adequate scope to improve the effectiveness of central planning in health sector, particularly medical care, nutrition, family planning, sanitation and water supply, etc. The health care professionals can contribute their might to make India a healthy, fit and economically viable country besides improving her image in international level.

The story of evolution of Police in India is also a long one and dates back to Vedic period. Manu, is regarded as the first law maker recording the principles of civil administration. The *Rigveda* and *Atharva Veda* are the first authorities to describe crime and punishment methods in India. Description of police force activities of those days is also available in our ancient records like Sanskrit drama *"Mruchha Katikam"* by Sudraka, *Sakuntalam* by Kalidas, *Arthasastra* by Kautilya, etc. The principles and practice of criminal investigations, punishments, vice control devices, spying including woman spies, rewards to loyal and good workers, and many other police activities of that time are found in ancient literatures. The Mughal period has introduced the system of revenue collection through agencies like *Zamindari* system. Akbar appointed provincial *Subedars* and the policing of big towns was managed as per law book

"Ain-i-Akbari" written by his Minister Abul Faz-al.

The beginning of modern police force system in India was basically to satisfy the imperialistic exploitation of East India Company which also used it to suppress internal security problems. The gradual but continuous reform, expansion and qualitative changes helped them to rule better and suppress anti-British sentiments of Indian mass. The British crown established special and expert control over the police organisations and ensured better service through them. The Sindh police force established by Sir Charles Napier on the model of Irish Constabulary was the first organisation of para-military nature and the experiment was followed in many parts of the country. The historic Sepoy Mutiny of 1857 made the Imperial Government to realise the inadequacy of existing police machinery and urgency of reorganising the same. The administrative exercises lead to drafting and enacting of Indian Police Act in 1961, which forms the corner-stone of the police administration in India even today. With series of changes and reforms in respect of personnel policy, *modus operandi* and criminal procedures, the police organisations in India have seen centuries of ups and downs, the major and significant changes of which have come after political independence of the country in 1947. The growth of population, rise in crime rate and deteriorating law and order situation have exerted pressure on the horizontal and vertical growth of police forces and development of armed and specialised police troops. The bulk of the police job is performed by the unarmed or civilian police where as their action is supplemented by para-military or armed constabulary in special emergency situation of break-down of law and order.

Rather than to describe elaborately the formation, command and control and other aspects of police forces, it is judicious to take an overall estimate of the "great police family" of the country. The whole of family is so vast that it is conveniently classified as Central Auxillary Agencies and the State Police Organisations. The Central agencies include special organisations like CIB, CBI, SPE, Para-Military Organisations such as CRPF, BSF, the Assam Rifles, RPF, CISF and India Reserves. Newer organisations like NSG and ITBP, specialised agencies like RAW are also included in this category. In addition there are large number of institutions run by Ministry of Home Affairs for training and performing jobs of special nature, like the Directorate of Police Wireless, National Police Academy, Central Institute of Criminology and Forensic Science, Indian Security Printing and Mints, Finger Print Bureau, etc.

The police organisation in the States comprises of civil and armed wings under the direct supervision of Home Ministry of the State Governments. The professional wing includes the CID, the Anti-corruption Department, the Railway Police and the armed police branches. Some States maintain the women police force, mounted police, the homeguard, the dog squad as their ancillary units.

The police activities have reached every village level. Because of pressing needs of constant policing in the rural areas, the rural police system has been developed in some States with small auxillary groups of ablebodied village boys with nominal training of drill. They form the village volunteer force, village defence parties, village resistance groups, village vigilance committee, etc., named differently in different areas and States. They are all included in the Great Police Family, the health needs of whom are considered in the subsequent chapters of this book. The magnitude is ill conceived without a proper and organised study and hence the field is neglected and under-estimated. But before going into the details of health problems of policemen of the country, a general over view of the role of police forces in India will be more appropriate.

Role of Police Forces in India--An Overview

The Indian Constitution with its unique characteristic of "Centralised Federalism" puts Police and law and order in the State list. The century old Indian Police Act (1961) has seen revolutionary changes in the formation, organisation and administration of the law enforcing agencies, be it political or social change. Under the provision of Government of India Act 1935, "Peace and tranquility of India or any part of thereof" was kept as a special responsibility of the Governor General.

His counterparts, the Governors also had a similar responsibility in the State. The system has not only drained out the State police budget on the maintenance of armed wing, but has forced the Central Government to raise and maintain specialised agencies of police to supplement the armed wing of the State Police Forces. Every civilised society needs adequate policing for maintenance of law and order and to protect the citizens rights. It is the basic requirement for a systematic progress and civic tranquility.

The very instinct of man as a social animal, no doubt makes him associated with his fellow beings, which is often dictated by the needs of social, urban or industrial life. Such an instinctual or mechanical human association under favourable circumstances may crystallise into "Crowd" with a higher degree of cohesion, reacting to common stimulus. Various factors may act as catalyst and the crowd may gain destructive impulse and create psychological tension. The steady gain in the momentum leads to a wild climax of public violence, the crowd being transmutated into a mob. The individual elements of "mob" are easily separable because of their lack of uniformity in back ground and general outlook. Whosoever may be the father of the mob, dissatisfaction, frustration and/or fanaticism are the mothers. The individual interest coerce to group interest which provokes the collective law breaking and public unrest.

The causative factors of the public unrest in the Republic India is fairly exhaustive which is even some times, a complete departure from its pre-independent counterpart. The organised as well as the unorganised sections of Indian society like students, labourers, Public Servants, *adivasis*, communalists, regionalists, language fanatics, even *Sadhus* and finally the policemen have indulged in acute and chronic public agitations of violent and non-violent varieties.

The postmortem study of public disorders reveals a deep seated malady which symptomatically manifests through processions, strikes, *bandhs, gheraos, dharanas,* hunger strike, go slow, pen down, *jail bharo, atmadaha,* etc. The vocabulary is rich in identical terminologies which may be adopted by the strikers as suitable to them and may culminate into any degree of law and order problem.

So far there is no known standardised and foolproof panacea for this social malady. The traditional and stereo type *modus operandi* of the administration in police operation of such situation is often purely symptomatic with an ill calculated dose. Imposing of Sec. 144, closure of institutions, clamping of curfew in selected areas, rounding up of miscreants are the time honoured methods of curbing disturbed law and order. At the cost of the process leads to secondary consequences due to superadded factors. Situation may demand undesirable and unpleasant drastic police operations like firing, teargas, lathi charges, etc. Final sequale of negotiations, withdrawal of cases, release of arrested persons may wipe off the story from public memory.

Like any disease, disturbances of public tranquility has its own incubation period and use of cops to combat the lawlessness is effective only at a particular stage. No relief is possible when tides in flood are high, till the water level chooses to subside on its own. Only a saint or a true statesman could perhaps spiritually disarm a violent communal mob. The convalescence is often peaceful due to traumatic experience of the unrest, though relapse cannot be ruled out. The outcome of violence like destruction to public property and harmonious civic life has far reaching implications of permanent or semi-permanent nature. It remains as the perennial virus in the area having its effect in the local political battles or group rivalry, like a bitter pill even if it is swallowed leaves an unpleasant taste in the mouth.

Scope of the Role

The para-military nature of the police forces is a paradox in itself. In defence services the group opposite is an enemy camp and its total annihilation with valour is a laudable objective. In case of any para-military organisation engaged in the mob control, the 'Opposite' group consists of citizens and it is no valour, even if one citizen has to lose his life. The scope of law and order so far as duties of police forces are concerned, it is not exhaustive with mob-dispersal or crowed control of a communal riots, student unrest or labour agitation. The long list of assignments like VIP security, guarding of residence of prominent VIP's, public properties and vital installations, search of unlawful arms and anti-social elements, public meetings, fairs and festivals, rehabilitation camps of refugees are only few to enumerate. Besides, the forces have well appreciated role in natural calamities, Republic Day celebrations, *bandobast* duty in all the general elections in the country due to the secular nature. Counter insurgency is also the familiar domain. The first agency to receive SOS from civil/State police is Central Home Ministry on the formers failure to handle a situation. It has stood as second line of defence to the regular armed forces of the Union in international border operations.

To kill people does not require that much of skill as is required to save people in the midst of violence. Here the dilemma of the police forces is that they have to accomplish a para-military job as well as of citizen with a difference. Paradoxically, its equipment is militaristic but its professional needs are ardently social and human. Here, while discussing the role of para-military organisation the old proverb "Every citizen is a police man without uniform and every policeman is a citizen with uniform" is to be remembered. Before stepping out for a duty as a policeman every member of police force must think that basically he is also one of the millions of civilian citizens but for the nature of duty he is assigned. Gone are the days when general public of lawful or unlawful gathering use to disperse just by arrival of Khaki clad policemen out of fear and the situation hence automatically controlled. Like a running vehicle stops not entirely by the breaks applied rather than partially because of its own weight. In the changed circumstances the police force has to gain the confidence of the public to operate effectively, rather than to represent as the muscle-man of the ruling political system.

As a law enforcing agency the police force is generally regarded as a part and parcel of the regulatory administration which should have little to do with the factual need of the public. This creates an aura of apprehension, anxiety and fear in the public. Police is immediately identified with law though they are responsible for safe-guarding the most basic elements of social life. On the nature of police only the general public may feel to the greater extent as to whether the Government is by men or by law.

The need for a central police organisation in a changed society rests on the failure of old Colonical district based muscle oriented police organisation, which is too rusty to be geared to the new tasks and roles. The political masters have equipped the police forces to defend *status quo* and to preserve the dead wood of political organisation as an executive arm of the magistracy, which bears historical legacy of centuries. The back thrust of an advancing society with mounting consciousness of fundamental rights, wider political participation and rapid economic development, is received by the police forces. By adopting judicious and balanced attitude these ill equipped police forces take care of the sabotages of development. Effectivity of police force is judged from the achievement of political stability, Industrial security and building a society with on going process of Democratisation, Industrialisation and Modernization.

Role of Social Justice

A democratic or socialistic society like ours which conceded to its citizens the fundamental rights of equality and liberty presumes that the majesticity of law will be respected by one and all. But in the day to day life of a civilised human being, justice represents a sort of workable compromise between the interests of strong and weak. In the simple principle of humanism, the weak should be protected against strong. These two categories have to co-exist always in any socio-political system by virtue of accidents like birth, sex, physical and mental incapacity.

Inspite of clear provisions in Indian Constitution to Rights of Life, Liberty and Equality of all citizens without discrimination of caste, colour, sex and creed, the metamorphic social transformations have overwhelmed the traditional societies. In the post-independent decades, the crime data shows that a sizable portion of criminal population in India originate and belongs to the traditional Weaker Sections of the society.

Similarly, the victims of criminal assaults are mostly the weak and the poor, who for varying reasons are deprived of adequate legal protection. Like the communal virus, this is also prevalently operative in the marrow of our society. Many experiments have already been performed to uplift their social status like supplying of arms to Harijans in Bihar, and opening of separate Police Stations within the jurisdiction of the existing one for weaker sections in M.P. have yielded fruitful results.

A secular, wide based and decentralised police force, having an all India composition is expected to render valuable service in bringing a workable equilibrium in the anomaly full and disparity prone society. Police is the first and most relevant agency of striking out the balance of social justice. The other agencies like courts, the Bar, the voluntary agencies and the Parliament come into play subsequently. Despite all big sympathy and voluminous legislation for the weak and the down trodden, the police philosophy of law enforcement, which is conditioned by history, tradition and even training of police men, is narrowed down the Blue-books and grey folders of Justice.

The public at large, and Weaker Section, in particular in their turn have a very poor image of police forces and their professional performances. The threatening insecurity haunts their lives and naturally, they cannot accept a foreign force as their protector or benefactor unless he goes to convince them whole heartedly about his credentials. The disciplined forces work under a hierarchy of an unified command. Such a condition is not suitable for the force to take up various projects in the fields of health, education, prohibition, co-operative farming, housing etc. for the weaker sections of the society, bringing a hall mark of change.

The Weaker Sections of the society in free India have multiplied quite rapidly posing social threat to law and order of the country. The population pressure has negated the additional productivity achieved by the Five Year Plans. The galloping urbanisation and uncontrolled mass migration to the new townships have compounded the rise of the problem. The increasing concentration of semi-urban dwelling with its vast army of unemployeds, frustrated and vulnerable to exploitation are readily available as nursery plots of crime and lawlessness. A rational look towards this aspect of society will be a fair-deal at the heart of the matter, and eradication of the virus. Once this is achieved, the Police Organisation will win the heart of the people and be a real friend of the masses.

Role As An Effective Police Force

Selection of role is vital for survival and development of any individual or organisation. In the words of Fyodor Dostoevsky, "If one wanted to crush, to annihilate a man utterly, one need only give him work of an absolutely, useless and irrational character. The effectiveness of police ensures survival by maximisation of development. "Police State" has been the predecessor of "Welfare State". Even the best form of the Welfare States of Democratic and Communist varieties have not succeeded in de-policing their societies.

It should be first realised that the law and order enforcement is not an easy commodity to sell in any country. By nature of their task, a police force cannot expect universal support and passion to be shown towards them. On the other hand, how much mental capacity is required for the police men to understand that though he speaks with society's authoritative voice he is also a responsible citizen of the same society.

Lack of effectiveness in police force in any society is one of the heaviest liability which the ruler as well as the ruled can ill afford. Like the army the high state of morals has to be maintained and once ineffectiveness sets in, the consequent demoralisation of cops is the dangerous outcome. Paradoxically speaking, an ideal situation of effective policing renders the police organisation dysfunctional, just as the peaceful world cannot rid itself from armies and arms. The existence of a healthy police force is a pre-requisite for the developmental endeavours of the individual and the society. The absence of police or its effectiveness as a law enforcement agency is bound to cause social indiscipline, which once allowed must result in erosion of faith in the basic values of high order.

The students of Police Science are acquainted with the terminologies as "Police Excesses" and "Police Restraints". They are the subjective assessment of given situations in a contextual frame. The political nature of police effectivity is yet to be understood. If the police acts to destroy the very purpose of the political system, it is obviously ineffective. The senior police leadership is stigmatised because of the major mistakes of non-police organisation whom the former has been trained to respect and obey.

The changing pattern of law and order has further deteriorated by the facts that inadequate strength of police force leads to grappling with mounting workload, penal provisions and procedural bottle-neck impending the prompt and honest course of law in bringing the culprits to book, which still enlivens the historical image of "Colonial Barbarity". Lessons learnt from Assam and Punjab operations demand redrafting of charter of duties, role and jurisdiction for all para-military forces. The existing police philosophy in India takes a very narrow telescopic view of role of police forces which needs to be drastically reformed. Moreover, the image of police force is a double edged weapon, which blurs the visible action of the force in the eyes of society as well as professional estimation of a force member.

In order to build an image of an effective police organisation in the changing patterns of law and order the Police Force has to make the society feel that it is the only organisation which comes as saviour in the hours of crisis in the psycho-social front of common man as if the mountain has come to Mohammad. Hence, it is high time for the forces to change their attitude of providing symptomatic and purely temporary relief from the activities of political leaders of Opposition, youth leaders of Campuses, the leaders of the minority pockets, the trade union leaders in the industrial belt and other emotional groups. It is not completely meaningless to suggest a "Citizen Police" or a "Positive Police" role rather than to be "Professional Police". It can certainly develop a non-military, progressive, timely, need oriented outlook from the frame work of a disciplined secular para-military force, which is the organisational necessity. Hence, the role of the police force in brief can be appropriately defined like that of UNO troops, under its limited internal frontiers, to usher an era of negotiation, peaceful co-existence and tranquility in the years to come.

Finally, the police functions in a democratic society is a complex one. It is becoming an uphill task for the police force to hear the voice of the community at large, crying out for aid, relief or redress inequalities and infringement of basic civil rights, operating under severe constraints. This is a big task, particularly at a time, when it is collapsing in every sphere of activity. A well determined role for the police force is required for the survival of the democracy at large and the police forces itself in particular.

2

Special Problems of Men in Uniform

When a policeman kills a dacoit risking his life in encounter, the hearts of public woo too much for the dead dacoit. The incident is described in the Press as "fake encounter". But when the dacoit kills a policeman, no one has a word of sympathy. When he is severely injured and "breathing to live" in hospital, he does not draw any public visitor except his brother policemen. Sometimes the public condemns the action of policemen as foolishness, undue risking and the police department itself, describing it as bad operational planning, etc. This is the usual story the police has been hearing since centuries. After the climax of incidence or police action, the dust settles for the purpose of public tranquility but the reputation and image of police remains tarnished even after the peace has been restored. That is because the action of police is never appreciated as justified, inevitable or the demand of the time and situation. Police forces in India have been fighting an "Undeclared War" continuously. Any military campaign lasts for days or months. But police operations last for years together. Some parts of the country or the other always remain "hot spot" and country's police forces are over burdened with duties and hardly have to time to relax, rejoice, spend time, with family, attend to personal problems and most important of all, get proper treatment for their illness.

Taking the entire police community of the country as a whole, uniformed and plain clothes, armed or unarmed, general or specialised, State or Central, constitute a vast population of guardians of law, who do not even draw up sympathy from the public. The illness, injuries and health of their families constitute the enormous task, being managed by the medical set up of the respective forces. This is where the khaki clad policeman and white aproned medical men intermix. The two professions have been marching together in war and peace. The experience has been a happy story for both the disciplines.

A question often asked by many as to why should there be a special police hospital or police doctor at all ? Why can't their families draw their medical assistance from the available civil hospitals ? Are they different from general public ? The following paragraphs would explain it elaborately.

The concept of police hospitals in India is quite old. Presumably there used to be a separate group of doctors who used to look after the inmates of prisons, detainees, undertrials, political prisoners and those arrested under MISA, TADA, and DIR. The same doctors were used to certify death after executing capital punishment. As such these doctors usually do not have much work to do as he used to attend duties in civil hospital in spare time and the employees of jails, police, homeguard and allied offices use to take treatment from him because of acquaintance and proximity. Their services in jail were further extended to the police camps and the beneficiaries were naturally the camp dwellers. This system further lead to opening of full fledged special police hospitals in district police centres managed by staff deputed from the State health service cadre and budgeting from the police fund. Since the police camps are established at the outskirts of the city, the opening of medical aid centre for the population was justified.

There are as few other factors which contributed to the growth of police hospital system, some of them are discussed below :

(i) Policemen are citizens with a difference. They are specialised group for a special task. By virtue of their regimentation, their loyalty to the State has to be beyond doubt. These poilcemen in course of their duties are to act against the criminals, anti-social elements, extremists, gamblers, hoarders and so on. This puts their own security and the security of their family and children at stake. Hence, the police hospital facility is a measure to avoid security hazards for policemen and their families.

(ii) The civil hospitals are unmanageably crowded. The policemen have to be spared from their duty point by suitable reliever to enable the sufferer to report to doctor for treatment, which takes greater part of the day. Such arrangement cannot bring quick relief to the policemen for his early return to duty.

(iii) The doctors in civil hospitals have poor knowledge about the rigours of police life. They have no time to understand the stress and strain the policemen receive from their normal duties. For instance, even "shoe bite" is sufficient to hamper the duties of a young recruit or policeman. The civilian doctor disposes it to be a minor problem. This problem is overcome when the treatment is undertaken in departmental hospital with the medical officer conversant with police life, their training, sports and other professional hazards.

(iv) The police patients requiring hospitalisation are preferably admitted to police hospitals for obvious purpose of better security and privacy. Besides many of them require long hospitalisation after bullet injury, bomb blasts injuries, accidents, amputations and fractures, etc. The civil hospitals show reluctance for shortage of beds. These cases are better managed in own hospitals.

(v) The doctors working in civil hospitals are not conversant with the systems and procedures followed in police and para-military forces. Hence, the official documentation etc. are not possible by them. Besides, it is only the doctors posted in a police force who would visit to far-flung out-posts where companies or platoon strength force are deployed and complete the annual medical inspection of camp and give health education advices. Hence, the medical cadre in para-military police forces maintains the lifeline of troops in respect of health and moral.

(vi) The members of police forces are not allowed for "self-doctoring". On their illness, the arrangement of treatment is the job of his immediate commander. And the nature of illness, degree of severity and capacity to perform duty has to be officially reported to the administrative in-charge. Hence, the correlation between the medical branch and the administrative offices is not possible unlesss both of them are under common command.

The role of police force hospitals is discussed at length in a separate chapter. Hence, it is needed to highlight that departmental hospitals with well formed medical cadre is an asset in managing the health care affairs of the police forces. Unlike the civil hospitals, who may look after only the curative part, the police force hospitals have the broader horizon including health education, staff training, follow up, disposal through medical board and rehabilitation. The arrangements for higher treatment at advance hospitals, recommendation for financial and other assistance for such treatment, looking after the community medicine aspect of the camp and other day to day affairs are also done by the police force doctors. Hence, the concept of separate medical care system for the police forces has been the order of the day and would go a long way.

Among the central police organisations the Assam Rifles happens to be the oldest para-military force of the century. The medical cover to this force which has its deployment and operational activities in North Eastern States parallel to army units, was provided by army. Subsequently, the force recruited their own medical men to extend medical services in static head quarters and training centres, in addition to the help received from Army Medical Core. Hence, the force receives services from dual sources.

The second oldest C.P.O., is the Central Reserve Police Force (CRPF) which came into existence in the year 1939 at Neemuch in the Malva region of the then Madhya Bharat (Central Province) under the name, Crown Representative Police. Neemuch is a climatically healthy place with moderate climate and continuous blow of Malva breeze. It was then a small township and was historically famous for its old military cantonments and the oldest "Opium and Alkaloid Factory" of India. The old Cantonment barracks were occupied by the CRP, which had a role to help the Centre in combating disturbed law and order. The force was transformed to the present form, the Central Reserve Police Force after Independence. Neemuch had poor medical facility at that time and the force had to open up their own hospital in the campus to prevent their jawans visiting the town for medical treatment and get involved in crimes like opium smuggling etc. which was rampant there. This is how the Crown Representative Police hospital of Neemuch came into being and bagged the credit virtually as the first hospital of Central Para-military Forces. Subsequent expansion of CRPF and creation of BSF, ITBP and other forces, forced them to form the in-built medical set up in their organisation and established chain of hospitals on strategic points.

Although as human beings, the Police personnel are prone to any disease, there are a host of conditions which are occupationally peculiar to the men in uniform. As such there is no systematic scientific and statistical study of morbidity pattern of police forces as to know its improvement or deterioration. But on general observation some transformations over the old morbidity pattern of past decades is inevitable, due to improvement in general living standard, urbanisation, health consciousness and better medical facilities available to the forces and their families.

Disease is only the detectable part of a complex process in which socio-economic-environmental-bio-pathological processes are involved. It is like the tip of the "iceberg" visible to the observer but it is submerged portion is manifold bigger in magnitude. Every disease process has a pre-pathogenic (pre-Clinical) Phase, a pathogenic (clinical) phase and the post-pathogenic (recovery or convalescence) phase. Clinicians put due importance to clinical phase during which intensive treatment is instituted and recovery phase is left to the nature with discharge advise from the hospital. The pre-clinical phase is like the submerged portion of iceberg, bigger in extent, has greater impact on the society and individual's health but usually neglected. The medical care system must cover all the three phases and the "total medical care" must have preventive, curative and restorative approach.

In absence of proper scientific data it is hardly possible to comment on the special problems of men in uniform. However, the following empirical classification of illness can be suggested :

(i) **Stress Disorders.** The range is wide but organic diseases like hyper-tension, Ischaemic heart disease, acid peptic diseases and psychotic illnesses are prominent. Osteo-arthritis changes spondylosis and diabetes Mellitus, etc. can also be classified under this category.

(ii) **Climatic Hazards.** Clinical condition due to extreme climatic conditions, high altitude, mountain, sea, solar radiation etc., the mosquito, fly and water borne diseases, thyroid goiter, hyper flourination (flourosis) are all in this group. Deficiency diseases, nutritional diseases also find place here.

(iii) **Infective Disorders**. In a close community life communicable diseases by cross infection are common.

High communicability is the hall mark of camp life. Any infective process from common to rare ones can be traced in the Forces. Epidemics of hepatitis, conjuntivitis, cholera and typhoid have been noticed many a times. Other conditions worth mentioning are venereal diseases, tuberculosis, leprosy, dental diseases, food poisoning, etc. Incidence of seasonal common cold, viral fevers are same as general public.

(iv) **Injuries and War Casualties**

(a) Operational Group--This is the major group of police morbidity in which maximum loss of lives and loss of working man days are recorded. Bullet injury, bomb-blast injuries and burns and accidental injuries are common mishappenings the policemen are exposed to.

(b) Exercise and Sports Group--Training programmes, sports, ceremonial parade, etc. are the day to day affairs in police forces. Every man in the force is exposed to varying degree of exercise throughout his career. Hence, sports injury of any nature is expected due to exogenous and endogenous causes.

The classification is empirical and experience based. Many more elements which need inclusion constitute minor groups or limited to a specific group of policemen. Few examples would clarify. The men of CISF guarding Atomic Research Centre (BARC) are likely to be exposed to radiation hazards, in fertilizer plants to accidental poisonous gas leak, in opium and alkaloid factory, affected by the sedative effects of the opium vapour during the process of dehydration etc. There may be innumerable such examples but each group is too small that they do not qualify for general consideration. New medical syndrome like Acquired Immune Deficiency Syndrome (AIDS) is not yet reported from any police force personnel in India till close of the year 1992.

According to stray report available from the Madras city police hospital, the medical officers have listed 5 major ailments which the police personnel normally suffered such as alcoholic neuritis, hyper-tension, diabetes, respiratory infection (mostly caused by smoking) and peptic ulcer. The surveyor has felt the need of better facilities, specialist services and better quality drugs in police hospitals. He has stressed the need of the comprehensive plan for total health care coverage in view of occupational hazards to which the police men are subjected Psychological guidance, counselling and health education programmes would change the scenario of police morbidity supplementing the perfect public health measures.

The study of morbidity pattern of army, which may be some what relevant to the national level forces, is interesting. For army, health is a battle winning factor. During wars, the hospital admission of war casualties and other illness are disproportionately high in the later. Morbidity and fitness are the direct index of failure or success of implementation of public health services. During peace time, the hospital admission is dominated by communicable (infective) and non-communicable diseases. In the later group 10% of the cases are due to injuries (non-enemy action) and rest are due to stress disorders. Among the communicable diseases Tuberculosis causes the highest man power loss; the other prominent illness being venereal diseases, dysentry, diarrhoea, Malaria, ricketsia group of fevers, enteric fever, cholera, etc. Plenty of statistical data and scientific study of military hygiene reports can be obtained for compilation and research work.

The military statistical data cannot be disposed up as irrelevant and entirely academic. There are lot of informations that can be drawn which are educative and guiding factors for any force medical services. The following inferences are helpful in police force set up also--

(i) Illness and non-war casualties predominate the morbidity pattern in police forces like army.

(ii) The credit of substantial improvement of illness pattern goes to effective military hygiene.

(iii) The improvement in sickness in forces has added materially to the fighting efficiency of the troops.

(iv) The upkeeping of standard requires constant endeavour and there is always a scope for further improvement.

(v) Further improvement is possible if lessons are learnt from past mistakes and experiences.

(vi) Health consciousness by all members of force and their families is an inevitable requirement to maintain best hygienic condition.

(vii) The principle of "Prevention better than Cure" must be strictly followed under able guidance of specialists in community medicine with co-operation from all.

Inspite of striking resemblance in the life style and duties with army, the police forces have their own originality, limitations and constrains. The army is made to maintain better standard and status for obvious reasons, than any police force. But even if we overlook the differences in the emoluments, ration facility, provisioning of clothing, equipment and other minor perks and benefits which directly affects the men, there is a paradoxical difference in the living standard, nature of duties and the degree of exposure to the professional hazards. The Central para-military forces and State armed police are engaged in the job of law and order day and night. The army has to fight a war only once in an extreme emergency of international dispute. But the police forces are fighting an "Undeclared War" in the streets with our own people, not enemies. The war is continuous and year long. They are always on their toes to combat militancy. The policemen on duty are most prone to fall prey to the militant's bullet. The police casualties are heavy in the terrorist infested States and areas and increasing trend due to induction of sophisticated weapons such as rocket launchers, improvised explosive devices, grenades and remote controlled weapons by highly organised groups.

The extent of loss of lives of trained man-power runs much beyond description. During the last decade 1981-82 to 1991-92 the total number of policemen lost their lives in terrorist bullets, bomb-blast, communal riots and rallies is 7144. It is frightening to note that 4756 policemen died in last 5 years. The two major para-military forces of the country the CRPF and the BSF had the heaviest loss of 504 and 866 men respectively in the same period. Among the State police forces the State of Punjab had to grieve for 1096 men followed by Uttar Pradesh where 552 policemen sacrificed their lives while performing duties in the greater national cause. The figures of injured policemen are still greater. Unfortunately, the trend of injury and death of police personnel is increasing in alarming rapidity. In the year 1991-92 alone, if the number of policemen killed on duty of 12 top States of the country put together, more than 3 persons are losing their lives in the hands of terrorists.

On the face of such grave crisis to the protectors of law, there is crying need of an efficient medical care system equipped and trained enough to handle all types of injured and diseased and to function smoothly like a well oiled machinery. Besides, the police duty itself has enough of adverse effects on the health of policemen. Particularly, the stress disorders are the distresses directly due to the exigency of police duty. About 20% of the active man-power is rendered incapacitated directly or indirectly due to stress disorders in the forces. The working procedures of medical set up in the police forces is discussed in other chapters. The role of doctors in the community needs no elaboration to explain its vitality and utility. The noble concepts held at the time of planning are not translated to real practice. Hence in every stage the lacuna plague the system and defeat the purpose. The remedy for such sick system is to undertake a total overhauling and modernisation on war footing. This is the only way the nation can save the large toll of valuable trained police lives being lost mercilessly on the streets.

The police forces comprise a large category of policemen who have varying degree of difference in their working, life style than the main body of fighting strong masculine troops. Although constitute only minor groups they have their own standing problems and entity in the forces. One such group is the women wing of police. Now all the state police have added women elements to their troops specially homeguards and the unarmed constabulary. Among the Central para-military forces, the Central Reserve Police Force has been the torch bearer in this field, raising one full battalion of women troops, training them and put them on duty at par with their male counterparts. The Border Security Force has also announced to go for similar exercise and many State police armed wings are likely to follow in view of increasing demand of their services on the face of increased women related crimes in the country. Women have also entered in large number as regular members of army, navy and air force in clerical, medical, nursing, in education core and in ground duties in air force. The number of women members in the clerical grade of police organisations is also sizable. A discussion on health problems of the fair-sex will be the most fair deal here.

Medical Problems of Women Police Force

India is one among the countries who are late to enrol women into the traditionally male police world. The Americans did it in 1911 and London police in 1915. Germany commissioned the first female in European Continent in 1918. The national cadet corp is first to impart combatisation training to school and college girls followed by some para-police organisations like the Home Guards. The need of women policing was felt in the rise in the involvement of more and more of women in criminal activities and other sensitive duties like procession, *satyagraha*, *dharna*, etc. The State police use to engage their women constables in jobs like house search, frisking of women passengers in air ports, catching women involved in smuggling, drug trafficking, immoral trafficking of girls, unlawful sex scandals and the most important in international espionage.

At the national level, the CRPF is the first para-military force to raise a woman battalion. The success story of the troops in handling law and order situation has been appreciated at Government and social levels. As per an old saying, "one experiment convinces the doer, where as ninety nine more are required to convince others". Hence, the experience of women battalion performances is too short to be evaluated for its classic value. Now since other forces have also put their women batallions on road test, the future workers will be in better position to assess and comment on utility in the new social trend. Ethically, equal opportunity cannot be denied to the fair-sex as the rapid social change has obliterated the sex boundaries. The degree of risk involved in the type duty they are asked to perform is summarised as under--

(i) Policing of social, religious and political assemblies where a large crowd of women and children is expected. This involves long hours of duty in the madding crowd and stampede. Women police workers are in extreme tension in the face of the mob.

(ii) Provision of escort and search of female detainees in police *hazat*, hospitals and court of law. This duty identifies the female police workers in public and likely to be the target of criminals and terrorist groups in her private life.

(iii) Interrogation of women involved in sex offences, smuggling, child lifting, criminal abortion, immoral trafficking of women, etc. During these riskful duties women police force have to tolerate slangs, vulgar comments, life threats and bribery offers from the affected parties. It produces plenty of mental stress.

(iv) Launching Public Relation Programmes to improve police image in public. Helping enrolment of women candidates in army and para-military forces.

(v) Collection of intelligence on women related crimes and helping the Criminal Investigation Department (CID) of police.

Although the job is hazardous, the performance of the women police force in the last three decades have encouraging track record, attracting more women candidates from all strata of society to join the challenging job. But all said and done, unfortunately, a woman is a woman. The managers of police force know where lies the limitations. Although by all humanistic approach, they are treated at par with their male counter parts, they differ anatomically, physiologically, have different epochs of biological life cycle than man and have severe socio-familial limitations which forbids the development of full activeness and dynamism required for a successful police career. Some of these aspects are discussed here.

(a) *Social Aspects*--The age old Indian tradition puts Indian women in many social roles such as daughter, bride, wife, daughter-in-law, mother, grand-mother and so on. The education imparted to her may help in shaping her life style but mostly loses productive utility after marriage unless the family, specially her spouse, is broad minded and accommodative. Even taking up of a civil job is sometime not allowed in the new environment despite qualification and eligibility. In such a situation, the entering to police job is not at all possible after marriage, more so as the job is looked down in the society. If she takes up police job before marriage her salability in marriage market is slashed down drastically. The girl has to cross many hurdles and be bold enough to severe worldly relations to enter the challenging police world. This great transition from one world to another needs enough of mental make up to adjust. The failures to adjust not only ruins her career but her future life also.

(b) *Anatomical and Physiological Aspect*--Structurally the woman is designed for taking active part in the reproductive process of human race. The act of "Child Bearing" is her bonafide functional responsibility which her male counter part cannot share. The post-delivery child care also falls on her shoulders, naturally. Of course, others can help her on this stage to some extent. Such conditions greatly interfere with the normal police duty of women. The limited period of maternity leave covers only a small part of the entire process. The commanders feel inhuman to put a pregnant woman or infant caring mother to on active duty. Such limiting factors are detrimental to the police career of women.

(c) *Biological Life Cycle*--The biological life cycle of a woman largely comprises of her menstrual, marital (Sexual) and reproductive lives. But the functional aspect is not limited to "child bearing and child rearing" only. The woman has other medical aspects influencing her police duties. The tension full menstrual cycles, high incidence of abortions and post abortive complications, pinch of separation from family, spouse, children, disruption in conjugal life, unsettled family life, worries of children education and a host of socio-medical problems affects her devotion and sincerity to police duty. Hysteric, maniac and other psychological problems, other stress disorders like hyper-tension, divorce and suicidal attempts have been commonly observed among police women.

Stress has been the root cause of menstrual and leucorrhoea problems. Chronicity of such conditions lead to chronic back-ache, urinary infection and other disorders. The incidence of hyper-tension, acid-peptic diseases, loss of appetite and subsequent sequel like general weakness, anaemia, lack of interest in surroundings, insomnia, irritative and obsessive behaviour, melancholic attitude, etc. are seen out of stress complications. The release of stress hormones like catecholamine, glucagon, cortisol and growth hormones is increased and all these have antagonistic action to anabolic effects of insulin. As a result the level of blood sugar tends to rise in stressful situations and when it exceeds the tolerable limit, the person gets diabetes mellitus. These diseases are of chronic nature and long standing treatment is required. Irregularity in treatment worsens the condition. Regular treatment and check up are not possible in the life and situation of armed forces member. To prevent the problems the police woman needs social, physical, psychological, emotional and health adjustment. The unit and subunit commanders of woman troops have to devote time, understand their problems, apply managerial skill and have human approach to solve the problems. The relevance of posting specially experienced doctors to the woman unit increases manifold than to the male units.

Exercise and Sports Related Health Problems

The police forces endeavour all through their service career to maintain ideal physique and sound mind. For this, regular physical exercise in the form of parade, sports, games, etc. are part of their regular and routine life. Every member of the force is given equal opportunity to take part in the regimental and athletic activities, annual refresher course, route march, cross country race, annual firing practice, besides the daily morning physical training schedule. It helps them to keep their body fit and mind alert, a sense of youthfulness, agility and promoting efficiency in the police duty. For every police man *Fitness is his Bread and Butter.*

Age is one of the most important determinant of sportsmanship, the other major factors being nutritional status, growth and genetic constitution. From childhood to old age, all stages of life requires exercise and sports allowing reasonable consideration for degree of severity and expectation of performance. The recruitment in police forces is allowed only after attaining the age of 18 years. At this age the candidate can show impressive sports performance to the recruiting team, if he had enough scope for coaching and practice in the school and junior college stage. The constabulary which are drawn mostly from the rural population and from lower socio-economic group attend the local village schools where the basic infrastructure for developing athletic talent are not available. The State or Central Government has established regional sports centres where the talented candidates from different sports groups are picked up and allowed to develop proper skills.

The adolescent age of boys and girls is the age of peak performance production in majority of sports events. At this stage the life reserve capacity of man is abundant and proper scope can yield best result. With the development of aging process, the physiological parameters tend to decline and the exercise capacity, muscular strength and stamina which show slow deterioration and reduce the performance. Obeying the natural physiological laws for a sports-man is binding, as crossing the limitation may be catastrophic, particularly in competitive sports. The scientific assessment of skill, endurance, strength and flexibility of body of a particular player at a particular age can help in determining his suitability to perform, although the degree of adoption varies. But for few exceptional cases, the body adaptability has limited scope to comply the increasing work-load incurred in sports activity.

Keeping the age factor in mind, the physical fitness of a sports-man depends upon his exercise tolerance, maximum aerobic power (endurance), maximum anaerobic power capacity, muscular strength and neuro-muscular co-ordination (reflexes). Body weight, obesity, alcoholism, smoking and nutritional status have their own impact on the overall fitness of the performer. Hence, the improvement of physical fitness comes from--

1. General physical, social and mental well-being.
2. Degree of self confidence.
3. Starting age and scope to exhibit talent.
4. Sound neuro-muscular co-ordination.
5. Absence of fear, depression in failure.
6. Adequate adaptability to stress and strain.

The opinion and advice of sports medicine expert is desirable at every stage of sportsmanship. Many important events in life like surgical operation, accidental injuries, evidence of major illnesses like coronary heart disease, diabetes, bronchial asthma etc. severely affect the sportsman's way of life. Specially, the sports--women who have the physiological approaches of life such as puberty, menarchy, pregnancy, delivery, puerperium and menopause, effecting their sports performance and career. Other influencing factors in a woman's life are marriage, child-care and social attitude, which are not only limiting but terminating effects on her sports life.

The common sports injuries occur due to lack of knowledge of rule of game, leading to wrongful performance, inadequate training techniques, equipments and knowledge to avoid mishappenings on performance and carelessness on the part of the players. In police forces, where the policemen are made to take part in various sports and games they suffer from many defects and deficiencies. Some of them are elaborated here--

1. Inadequate practice in school age in rural background, and hence games to recruits and constabulary are thought as punishment.

2. Improper and inadequate coaching facilities with not-so-efficient coaching staff.

3. Aptitude or liking of a particular individual is not respected and they are compelled to take part in games at random and asked to produce result.

4. Practice with improper sports-kit, unsuitable protective garments, ground, track, mattresses etc.

5. Exposure to un-accustomed environment without proper aclimatisation, poor light, poor living conditions and inadequacy of nutritive value of food served to sportsmen.

6. Bad habits like smoking, alcoholism, drugs to improve performance, to reduce weight, unjudicious use of ready energy agents like glucose, steroid, and immoral activities like womanising.

7. Improper understanding among players, over enthusiastic desire to reach the top and lack of commonsense in crucial moments of game.

8. Discontinuity in practice or preparation for competitive sports on operational commitments.

9. Lack of proper incentives to best performers and depression among the losers.

These are only a few aspects of the problems in police forces which prove dangerous to health, produce injury of any severity, even fatal. The direct and indirect cost of such injuries cannot be calculated. The loss may be irrepairable and may leave permanent deformity. Hence, any sports injury should not be treated as negligible and complete treatment must be instituted in all cases. In deserving cases, rehabilitation measures must be taken. The players suffer maximum sports injury from games like football and gymnastics, where as the least injurious effects are from Tennis and cross-country race, according to a study by A.B. Corrigan (1968). Further, the commonest site of injury are knee (23%) and back (16%), while the trunk and head (0.5% each) are least affected.

Most of the injuries worsen due to non-availability of timely medical aid and proper sports medicine expert who may be capable to assess the severity and suggest measures to arrest further damage. The speciality of sports medicine is not included in the under-graduate curriculum of medical colleges in India. At the post-graduate level, only limited centres impart training to doctors sponsored by different government departments of the centres and various State Governments. Although sports and other exercise oriented training programmes are part of life in the Indian police forces, the culture of providing scientific medical coverage to the exerting sports-persons has not been developed. Hence, an important aspect of the sports management is over-looked.

The 'over-use injuries' or 'over-training performance' injury constitute the major group of sports injuries occurring in all types of sports. The occurrence of such injuries result from a number of factors including avoidance to pre-course medical fitness of the player, disregard to medical opinion and compelling and adamant behaviour of coaches and sports officials without foreseeing the un-toward consequences. Moreover, there is a general tendency of public as well as the sports administrators to blame the player entirely on poor performance or sustaining injuries, which affect the moral of the team and individual players. The obsessive tendency of the athletes to continue the activity and take part in competitive sports creates further problem to managers, doctors and the patient himself. The common factor in all over-use injuries is the repetitive micro-trauma at an anatomical site on continued performance even after injuries, causing further damage to the extent of tissue sickness.

The prevention of most of the injuries caused by sports and rigorous exercise can be possible by elimination of certain defects in sports management and systematic approach to the problems. Some of the measures suggested are listed below--

1. Thorough medical screening and aptitude testing before putting a young man to participate in a particular sports item. Diagnosis of angenital mal-

formations and systemic pathology which may limit activities or may bring adverse consequence must be done carefully.

2. The trainers should develop human approach to the injury prone athletes and physical conditioning should be carried out by gradually intensified exercise schedule.
3. Sports physician with familiarity with bio-mechanics of sports and better knowledge of the patho-physiology of over-use sports injuries should be engaged in the duties to cover the active programmes, with physical presence in the stadium.
4. Health Education imparted to players on personal hygiene, safety measures, limitations and adverse effects of drugs, alcohol and smoking must be a part of the training.
5. The deviation of game rules must be strictly guarded by the umpirical staff and supervision.
6. Freedom from domestic, economic, and administrative strain must be ensured to expect better performance. Proper rest, home-visit, entertainment and nutritious diet with required calorific value must be provided.
7. Any report on health and injury of the sports persons must be dealt with due consideration to his next competitive performance. Psychological fear and tension must be excluded.
8. The reasons for deterioration of performance and modalities to improve must be considered by board of experts, including sports medicine specialist. The sports doctor if so desires, may seek the help of any other specialist to decide the line of action on particular case.
9. Hasty return to full activity as well as very long period of rest in pretext of sports injury must be avoided to save deteriorating effect on the career and performance.

10. Proper physio-therapy and rehabilitation must be planned.

The health of female participant of sports is also of special significance. When members of the fair-sex enter the sports arena, extra precautions are required to be taken because this category of sports persons are more prone to injuries, not entirely due to poor conditioning or training. The advocates of feminocracy will not excuse me if I brand them as inferior sports persons, but their anatomical structure make them vulnerable to sports injuries, most of them occurring at knee and ankle areas. Severe fracture and head injury in sports-women are virtually unknown as games like football, boxing and wrestling are still not so popular among them. The breast and reproductive organs are also prone to injury from minor problem like rubbing of under-garments over skin of these parts to harmful consequences in her reproductive and conjugal life. Active sports during the first trimester of pregnancy may lead to miscarriage and the rise in uterine height and the weight of the foetus in later months compels the player to stay back from field. The emotional change, anxiety and fear during pregnancy, menstrual period, dysmenorrhea and meno-pause affect the performance in field and track events. Her participation in less exerting exercise programmes depends as to how she maintains her functional fitness, body shaping, flexibility and reflexes. Some of the best performances in sports-women are recorded in their post-menstrual phase. But no girl should be forced into or prohibited from competition during the period of menstruation. Police women need to adopt to family welfare measures to avoid unwanted or untimely pregnancy in order to upkeep their sports and service record.

The description of individual and group of sports injuries, their diagnosis and specific treatments are avoided purposely in this section. Such elaboration would have made the subject lengthy as it is beyond the scope of this work. The matters are in relevance to the police force activities, although much are still to be done. The physicians, psychologists, educational philosophers and physical educationists are required to conduct research as there is much scope to improve the health standard of sports-men and thereby the sports, at every stage.

3

Basic Needs of A Police Force

Ask any police trainer, 'What a policeman should be like?' The answer is invariably 'He should be like a policeman', or at best he would say, 'a policeman should be physically fit and mentally alert'. In other words, the policeman should follow what the fixed pattern of code of conduct, regimentation, traditions and norms his predecessors have set, besides being tough in physique, sound and watchful in mind, sensible to surroundings, reactive to stimulus and responding to call of duty. But to keep a policeman in such a fit and prepared condition, or the policeman to preserve the police dynamism in him, the basic needs of a policeman must be fulfilled. The factors eroding the standard, deteriorating the health and moral and bringing adverse effect on the disciplinary control of men, must be eliminated. Some of the salient basic needs are discussed here.

1. *Food and Nutrition.* The State Police Forces have troops mainly drawn from the State only but in the national level police forces, an all India composition is maintained. The food

habits of the people of different States and regions varies. But since they share the common kitchen food in the police barracks, it may not be possible to cater to the choice and taste of each individual force members. Inspite of that, the menu should be planned in such a way that all category persons get their choice of food sometime in the month or fortnight. Food is not only a basic need of man or *sipahi*, good food can be one of the attractions to the new recruits and constabulary to continue in the force, since they are drawn mostly from lower socio-economic group and standard of food is not upto mark in their houses. Nearly half of life's struggle is for procurement of food and half of individual's earning is spent on food. It is only good food that would build a good policemen, as *'soldiers March on their Stomach'*.

Besides the type of food, proper nutritional value and calorific yield of such food should also be considered. The food must contain all essential ingredients like carbohydrate, fat, protein, water, mineral and vitamin yielding sufficient energy to enable the person to perform physical and mental work, to repair tissues damage by normal wear and tear in his body and also leave sufficient residue in the lumen of small intestine to stimulate proper peristalsis, helping proper evacuation of bowel. The basic principles of sanitation must be followed for cooked and uncooked food articles and must be kept in highest standard to avoid any contamination, water borne diseases, food poisoning, etc. When the policeman is admitted in hospital he is supplied free food from hospital kitchen at government expenditure. But ordinarily he meets the expenditure of his own food which is partly compensated by ration money. Due to rising prices, at times the standard of food has not been maintained. The main cereal is procured from the depots of Food Corporation of India at Government fixed price but the vegetables, non-vegetarian articles and condiments are procured from open market. The system is satisfactory but needs constant vigil to prevent fall in standard while in the hands of greedy Mess Managers.

2. *Housing and Environment.* The accommodation should be proper, adequate and decent. It should also be complete

with water supply, electricity, drainage system and ventilation with mosquito proofing. In the State police, the *kotwali* and district police centres accommodate their men in family quarters and single men dormitaries. But in training centres, armed police wings and the central para-military forces accommodate most of their men in barracks. The permanent stations have limited family accommodation for staff. In police forces who frequently move from one "hot spot" to other on the demand of State Police administrators are housed in temporary settlements like old barracks, school or college buildings, club houses or in tents in open grounds, as it is seen in Central Para-military Forces.

Men returning to barracks after long hours of duty at odd time of the day, deserve some basic facilities like continuous water supply to bath and clean their clothings soiled with sweat and dust. Each barracks should be attached with kitchen to serve hot food and a calm and quiet environment for taking rest. Hygienic maintenance of barracks with rows of shade giving trees around, to keep the environment cool and fresh, fool-proof system of disposal of refuges and well maintained lawns and gardens around may increase the dignity and grace of police life. Due to rapid expansion of troops in changing law and order situation, it is not possible to house all men under built up accommodation. In such cases, canvas accommodation is provided. Canvas is not capable of protecting the inmates from extreme heat of summer, cold of winter or rains. Moreover, it faces damage in cyclone and fire. In recruits training centres and duty battalions the tentage camp sites should also be provided with other basic facilities. Cases of rhinitis, pharynsitis, bronchitis etc. are common in cold climate and heat-stroke in hot summer among the tent dwellers. Men get parasitic intestinal diseases as they are close to the soil.

Whatever may be the state of housing, supply of safe drinking water is a common demand among men. Proper arrangement saves men from taking water from contaminated sources and get water borne diseases.

3. *Exercise*--Exercise has been a way of life in the police forces. Exercise out of the normal duties, PT, Parade and training

courses is supplemented by special exercise programmes like jungle camp, commando course, rock climbing, mountaineering and sports. The programmes are made in such a way that every member of police forces is exposed to regular schedule of exercise so that he keeps himself fit and tough throughout the career. As the age advances, the courses should be of less strenous nature. It is part of their career planning. Improper planning leads to post exercise hazards like obesity, arthritis, diabetes, etc. Hence, every individual must be meticulously screened before putting him on vigorous exercise programme considering his age, associated diseases like hearing or visual impairments, hyper-tension skeletal deformity, systemic cardiac or respiratory diseases. Once the policeman develops such problems due relaxation from strenuous duties or exemption from night duty, route march, long driving, hill driving, etc. can be recommended. Graded *yoga* exercise can be prescribed in some cases. The problems related to exercise and sports are described in other chapters.

A good exercise and duty schedule keeps the policeman busy and tiring and the beneficial effects of such situation in police force set up are many. He can overcome monotony and freedom and he gets good appetite and good sleep. All these keep the policeman free from mental worries and disease free.

4. *Rest*--Rest is essential after hard work for regeneration of working capacity. It includes both physical and mental rest. Every policeman after certain hours of duty must be allowed to take complete rest in peaceful atmosphere and healthy surroundings. It is a debatable matter as to how much of rest should be allowed to the members of armed police forces on active duty. Unlike the civil jobs, the policemen or the armed police forces have to undertake mostly standing on sentry duties, parade, running, exercises, route march, patrolling, etc. which are strenuous and involves unlimited duty hours. In a normal working individual, it is generally, advised to divide the day of 24 hours to three equal parts, 8 hours each. Out of this one part (8 hrs) should be spent in for hardwork, another part in light or moderate work and the third part should be devoted for rest. Since the job of a policeman is by all means

tougher than non-combatised civilians, he cannot be prescribed anything less than this. As a matter of principle his hard work period be partly converted to light work but the period of rest cannot be reduced. Out of the restful eight hours, atleast 5-6 hours must be spent as bed rest for muscular and mental relaxation. A substantial part of the day must be allowed for his recreation or entertainment.

The policeman or members of armed forces get monotonous of their routine nature of work. The intermittent diversion of mind in entertainment, work of choice or changed nature of work must be allowed. The individual may allot his own time for any personal hobby or extra curricular acitivities. Men with family may find great solace in spending time with children, taking them around to sight seeing or picnic spots, movies, circus, *mela*, market or shopping to buy personal school requisites, social visits, etc. Members of police force must be prohibited from taking the help of drugs, alcoholic beverage or any other measure for getting good sleep. Such abuse may be habit forming and addictive. As a matter of practice, ideal programme of intermittent work relax-sleep schedule is not being possible in rotation in the working pattern of police forces. There is no fixed hours of duty and in heavy operational areas men are put on duty upto 10-11 hours continuously. And due to various reasons, the same troop is again put on duty. The reasons range from exigency of duties, sports, administrative and office duties, ceremonial parade or natural wastage like death, retirement and resignation. These posts continue to be unfilled for months together, causing extra burden on the remaining troops. Such situation reduces the scope of allowing full rest to all men after hard work.

5. *Games and Sports*--Every member of police force should take part in some games and sports activities. Such activity not only exposes hidden talent in sports field but promotes mutual co-operation, team spirit and closer friendship among members of police force who are drawn from the various socio-economic strata and diverse geographical natives. It should be part of the daily life of a policeman in addition to the regimental column drills. Jawans and JCOs (Junior Commissioned

Officers) or SOs (Subordinate Officers) who are put to office jobs, develop sedentary habits unless they are put to regular exercises through games. Even in middle aged police officials, regular physical activity helps to avoid deposition of fat and ill-shaping of the body structure. It should be planned in such a way that every member gets ample chance to take part in the competitive and practicing games. The commanders of the police battalions use this as the best mode to get the men tired and get good sleep at night without drug or alcoholic drinks. Some games being seasonal, the players should be allowed to take part in multiple games. Some persons show extra interest in a particular game and attain professionalism. Scientific evaluation by trained sports medicine doctor on stamina, performance and scope of improvement for a candidate to a particular game, even particular post in a game are being followed in the national and international sports centres. Such practice may be required for making sports records. But here in the troops, the aim is to give all men equal opportunity to play game, needless to say that it is in the true spirit of game.

Modern sports require lots of paraphrenalia like fields, tracks, sports kits, equipments, sports suits and so on, which are expensive and cannot be catered for all men. Hence, traditional sports like *kabaddi, khokho* and yogic exercises should be played which are possible even in field areas and small detachments. Unarmed combat exercises are also practiced as regular sports in absence of sports gadgets.

6. *Family Life*--The service in armed police of the State and civil police are mostly restricted to the State boundaries. Hence, it is only on rare occasions the troops are out of the family station for long duration. But the situation is altogether different in Central para-military forces. It is in some forces now, a few family stations have been established where the limited family accommodation, houses the permitted families. But such facility is so meagre that only 10 to 12% of entire armed police population can avail at point of time. Hence, but for those handful privileged persons all others leave their families and children in their native villages and home towns and serve in far flung places, leading a 'forced bachelor' life.

Naturally, the permission granted to families is only for a specified period, vacating and making it available to next man in waiting. Because of sudden movement of troops, lack of similar infra-structure in the field areas, increased risk of militancy, etc., it is not possible to allow all men of armed forces to keep their families with them. In some semi-permanent locations, the persons are allowed to enjoy family life on extreme compassionate ground on hired accommodation outside the camp.

Family is that social institution which provides priceless happy returns in life. It makes the perfect balance sheet of family economics, caters food of choice in time, creates healthy environment for development and education of children, ensures sexual satisfaction and so on. All these gives the policeman satisfaction in life which enables him to perform his duty perfectly, keeping him healthy and fit and inhibits him from indulging in any unlawful activity or to commit any crime. The emotional and sentimental element due to separation from family is eliminated. Their attachment to children is kept intact. The repeated request to proceed on leave by arranging fake telegrams and letters with messages of death and illness are avoided when they are with family. There have been number of cases in police forces when mental and emotional disturbances are noticed both in men and their families. Separation due to which also creates other social problems like adultry, prostitution, diverse misunderstanding in couples and perversion, like masturbation, lesbianism, etc. Needless to emphasise that family life is one of the most important basic need of men in police forces, the hard fact not realised by others not facing similar condition.

7. *Dress*--It is the dream of a dutiful devoted policeman to be well dressed, which gives him a good personality, smartness and the pride of police profession. It also reminds him of his identity and sanctity of police duty. The troops with well fitting, well washed, well-ironed and well maintained uniform have the best turn out and also have reasonably good health. The most vital role played by the soldier's dress is the development of his consciousness about his own physique,

figure and fitness. The seasonal clothings of winter or hills and snow prevent exposure to cold, frost bite, etc.

8. *Welfare*--Welfare is a broad term, covering a wide range of subjects. It is the basic factor to keep the moral of the force high. A Commander can motivate his soldiers to go to war only if he has looked after their best welfare all through the peace time. In a para-military unit or peace formation, there are three most important officers who are directly responsible and involved in the welfare of men and their families. Firstly, the commanding officer, looks after the timely payment of dues, liberal grant of loans, grant of leave and other service benefits. Secondly, the Subedar Major, who forms the link between the lower ranks and the supervisory officers. He reflects the feelings in the lines to the brass board offices. And lastly, the medical officer. The doctor and his team of para-medical staff look after the sick men and their families. Hence, hospital becomes the centre of welfare activities and medical staff provide immediate relief to distressed police personnel and their families. The separated families are comfortable in presence of medical cover in absence of the head of the family. Employment of dependents on the casualty or invalidation of the bread earner of the family has the best sort of welfare the unit can undertake, supplementing the earning of the family through work in the central fabrication centres is a regular way of life in Central para-military force group headquarters.

When the troops are out of headquarters on duty, the medical coverage to their families is one of the best form of welfare. The sympathetic attitude of doctors and helping gestures of other officers and staff consoles the families and boost the moral of policeman on duty.

9. *Reward of Good Work*--It is already discussed that the job of a policeman is one of the oddest in nature. The police performs one of the most thankless job in the society. There is hardly anybody who realises the gravity of his work, which they do by playing hide and seek with the hard-core criminals and terrorists at the risk of their own lives. The society or government has nothing to give in return except the occasional

rewards from the department or the government. The rewards may range from written appreciation, commendation entry in service book, cash reward and in exceptional nature of work and bravery, the police medals. Such enouragement and incentives are essential to boost the moral of police force for remarkable work in operational sports and other fields. Apart from senior officers, for good work goes a long way in the service career of a policeman.

10. *Medical Cover*--The medical cover is the life-line in the working system of any police force. This book is entirely devoted to the description of role of medical branch of Indian Police Forces. Hence, the subject is dealt in length in all other chapters. It is the key-word of welfare, moral and comfort in the police forces. Marching hand in hand in war and peace, the doctor is the friend and philosopher to the troops.

11. *Entertainment*--The arrangement of entertainment and recreational facilities is the integral part of the system in any army, police or para-military unit. Such arrangements play a vital part in maintaining healthy mind in the monotonous work of police life. Men in far-flung areas, separated from family and friends should have some mental recreation after hard-work. In the base camp family stations, the men and their families all enjoy the recreational programmes, arranged regularly. The range of such programme is wide such as Movie screening, regular T.V. programme, video picture show, newstrack, sports and video games. They are treated as the modern day entertainments. But old and not-so-old sources like Radio, Tape Recorder, Stereo, newspaper, magazines, etc. also serve to enrich their knowledge, passtime and break the monotony. Some find pleasure in performing arts like drama, variety show, indoor games like cards, carroms, etc, whereas some draw pleasure out of Annual Day mela, singing *bhajan* and playing *dholak* in *mandir*. There are also men who are fond of good-food, dress etc. and eagerly wait for *barakhana* evening. There are also exceptional talents in police forces as poets, painters, sketch-graphers, carricaturists, cartoonists and musicians. Even a regular mail service in the field areas serves as very important mode of keeping men jolly and cheerful.

During these programmes, educational films like health education, civic duties, traffic rules, family planning methods, etc. can be shown which can guide them in life to be good citizens. In family stations, films on vocational guidance, extra curricular activities, hobby and career planning can be shown for the benefit of children. Post retirement rehabilitation schemes would be of great interest to men on the fag end of their service.

12. *Children Education*--In the Central para-military forces, where the police forces spend most of the time in duty battalions, the children's education of men and officers suffer severe set-back due to frequent movements, change of school, syllabus, dress, medium of instructions and coverage of curriculum, etc. When the family and children are left in home-town or family stations, the children do not enjoy the supervision and guidance of father. The worries of the future of children compels the armed policemen to proceed on leave frequently, over-stay from leave or may finally decide to resign from the job or even desert the force. The problem has been partially solved by setting up of family stations, complete with Montessory School, Central School, local and municipal schools and ancillary services like school bus at nominal charges. In addition to the provision of government employees benefits like scholarships, tuition-fee, hostel subsidy and children education allowances, the forces have established chain of their own public schools, Industrial Training Institutes and have extended reservation in medical and engineering colleges at various parts of the country. This has assured the building of future of force members and relieved their mental tension and encourages them to perform their duties in hard areas.

13. *Leave and Vacations*--Spending of leave is one of the ways of relaxation for the men working far away from homes. Every year, casual leave for a fortnight and earned leave of one or two months are allowed to all members of Force. Such leave or vacation is essential as the men find change in monotony of routine life, meeting friends, relations, parents, families, kith and kin, negotiating marriage of self or other dependents, attending to landed or other property affairs. Leave or absence

from duty also helps in convalescing patients and removal from barracks during infective period after suffering from infectious diseases. On the event of any casualties in the family, he is granted leave on special compassionate ground with free travelling facility. The non-availability of leave due to exigency of service and operational commitment keeps him mentally upset and worried for his personal affairs. All men should be encouraged to go on leave arranging the programme in proper plan and thereby help them relieve his tension.

14. *Post Retirement Benefits and Rehabilitation Schemes*--Members of armed police forces who spend the best part of their lives in the service of the nation should expect fair deal from the employer such as governmental department. They expect to get a peaceful life after retirement through beneficial post retirement schemes. The benefits should not be restricted to financial gains, the range should be extensive such as allotment of plots, membership in self financial housing colonies, easy accessibility to ration and other commodities through public distribution system, facility of schools for dependents, vocational training for the retired and their children for self employment or part time engagement medical cover, etc. Police personnel after retirement can be re-employed in private guards and security jobs to have some handful income to meet the challenge of price rise. Since these persons are disciplined, they can take up civilian jobs of less laborious nature.

15. *Respect to Religious Sentiments*--The composition of police forces represents all States, religious, language and geographical areas. It is true in Central para-military forces where they are expected to be more impartial, secular and above the narrow consideration of caste and creeds in the public dealings. Inspite of these, the religious belief of every individual members are well respected. They are allowed to worship, pray and have faith in any God of his choice. The regimental centres have all religious institutions like Mandir, Masjid, Gurudwara, Church, etc. and men celebrate all religious functions collectively. Even after death, the funeral rite is performed as per the religion of the deceased policeman. The religious prayers and worship

have value in providing mental peace to the men. It should be duly regarded.

16. *Job Satisfaction*--Every worker needs job satisfaction which has several factors like congenial atmosphere in working place, job enrichment of the policeman's worklife and the motivation to work. The under-current of monotony and dissatisfaction in police job flows leading to lack of motivation and inefficiency, while satisfaction and job content produces maturity and efficiency. While police professionals are made to do any job at any point of time as a matter of compulsion, there is perceptible dislike of items such as domestic dispute, traffic control, handling of dead body, etc. Many surveys reveal that nearly 80-90% of calls received in police stations are related to miscellaneous non-crime work such as request to intervene domestic disputes, drive away animals causing nuisance, locate missing child, etc. Policemen are weary of attending such jobs and try to avoid, by-pass, delay or try to extract money from the public. Although the nature of job cannot be radically modified, the policemen should be persuaded that their job is meaningful to the society and their energy is well spent.

The effectiveness of inviting ideas from every employee on how to enrich job follows active motivation as the co-operation of all ranks in the force is required for a more satisfying job.

4

Manpower Planning and Police Health

The modern police forces are judged by their effective policing in the highly complex society. It has to face the multiplicity of functions, the increasing intensity of operations and wide spread geographical distribution of deployment of troops. In view of the increasing demand of police force deployment in a society with deteriorating law and order, the expansion of police forces and improvement of their quality of service are parts of their process of survival. To produce the right number at the right time, the government have to have a systematic approach in the framework of modern management science. This system covers the entire manpower planning which grossly includes proper recruitment, proper staff training, proper placement, career planning, job analysis and job incentive, etc. The policy planners of the police forces are satisfied with issue of circulars and instructions on the physical, educational standards for entry to various police forces. The few fixed criteria are for the policemen for "General Purpose". Gone are the days when the police duty use to be of very mechanical and routine in nature, where a semi-literate simple young man was able to deliver goods. Now the police job has many special areas where skillful manpower is required. Hence, the need for picking up young educated and moderately intelligent police recruits are the order of the day.

Basically, the policeman is expected to maintain peace in the community and this duty demands more of physical reserve than mental faculties. This impression puts education in a back-seat. Higher education has its own advantages in every sphere of police and personal life. But lessons learnt from country wide police agitation in 1979 is that it was the large number of well educated young constabulary gave leadership to agitating policemen, nullifies the concept of drawing highly educated persons in lower ranks.

There has been varying opinion on age of entry. At the constabulary level, the training is tough and long. The young flexible bodies would be more suitable hence the age group of 18 to 22 years with energy and drive to face the hardship is welcome. For higher rank entry such as Subordinate Officer or Gazetted Officer the educational and intelligence requirements are higher and the duration of physical training is shorter. In such cases, the candidates should not have attained the age more than 25 to 28 years.

Unfortunately, there is no personnel policy in many of our police forces. Since growth of forces are inevitable, they are anamalous and without any meticulous planning and management philosophy. The resultant complications are treated symptomatically without long term effects. There is no continual research and development activities or any such outfit to stream-line, rectify anomalies and implement clear cut government policy. Every year, thousands of vacancies are occurring because of "natural depletion" such as super-annuation, resignation, death, invalidation, voluntary retirement, transfer to other departments etc. But more number of vacancies occur suddenly on the sanction of new battalions. To replenish the regular depletion of strength and to supplement the force, every force requires on effective manpower planning cell who should look after the aspects like--

(a) anticipation of vacancies and measures to fill them up.

(b) development of manpower through proper training.

(c) aptitude testing for placement of the right man in right post.

(d) eliminating unsuitable unfit members through proper administrative and medical procedures.

(e) rehabilitation of rejected policemen, and

(f) motivation of defaulters.

The following paragraphs have the limited scope to deal with medical aspect of recruitment and health education in police forces.

One may ask what is the relevance of manpower planning in police forces to the health of the personnel ? The two have vital link. When new battalion or group centre is raised, the nucleus staff is drawn from the trained staff of existing battalions and units. As a result, the working population or the effective strength of the old units are thinned out. The functioning of the old units are severally affected. The left over manpower have to face the rigours of over-work leading to deterioration of health. The vacancies are not filled up till the new recruits complete their basic training which is of nine months duration. It is like the cancerous growth on any part of the body leading to general catchexia of the whole body. Such situation should be avoided for proper healthy development of the force.

Health Screening at Entry Point

The selection of future policemen is done by nominating the fittest and the best in the crowd, eliminating the undeserving lot. This is the entry point of men to the police profession. The health standard of future police force depends upon how thoroughly the recruitment has been conducted.

The criteria of physical and medical standards are already laid down in the statutory rules and orders. But for the minor variations for special category policemen, the enlightment standard remains more or less same in all forces as the basic aim is to accept the best as input to the uniformed community. Besides, the men of Central para-military forces like CRPF, BSF, Assam Rifles etc. are sometimes required to under-take combined operational exercises with men of State reserve police, provincial armed constabulary, special armed police, etc. The CPOs serve as the country's second line of defence. Hence, equally graded training, like army has to be imparted to these forces. For this reason there cannot be any compromise in the health standard of the para-military troops irrespective of their controlling ministry. A defence like preparedness is expected among the men of armed police forces throughout the year.

The tedious screening procedures in recruitment of police force have been designed to ensure proper elimination of clinically apparent unhealthy candidates and enlist only healthy and strong work force, which crystalizes to become actual guardian of security of the country. The executive and medical officers engaged in the task of recruitment may use their best judgment in final selection. Some of the general recruitment guidelines are common to all the State and Central forces, though the rules are framed by different government bodies at different time. Keeping in view the standard expected, the general growth and built of the State or region based on geographical and regional peculiarities, tribal community, etc. minor variations cannot be ruled out. Besides the enlistment team may refer to the latest amendment of rules and orders so as to give legal justice to the candidates. Some of the generai guidelines are listed below basically depicts the recruitment concept of Central para-military forces.

1. The first phase of recruitment includes taking of physical measurement of the candidate such as height, weight, chest, etc. Verification of age, educational documents, caste certificate etc. follows next. All these works are done by executive people and assisting staff. The doctor accompanying the team has also a role to supervise the work and rectify faulty measurement, etc. Besides, he can observe the general appearance of candidates, defective gait, deformity in limbs, incoherent talk, etc.

2. *The Measurement of Height*--requires careful consideration. The candidate is made to stand erect against the standard with feet together, the weight of the body thrown on the heels. His head, shoulder, buttock and calves should tower the stand. The chin should be depressed to bring the vertex of the head level under the horizontal bar. Height should be recorded to half centimeter accuracy.

The stature of a person is the first criteria after full growth which he attains by 20-21 years. If any candidate is below 20 years of age, he may gain height in future. Hence, the final measurement of height should again be done after the age of 22 years for entry into his service record and identity card. Hence, the measurement and recording of height should be done perfectly. Good height contributes to the personality of the troops which is an added advantage in duties like crowd control.

3. *The Chest Measurement*--is significant for it is an index of growth and developed musculature and respiratory status. A good chest measurement and adequate expansion capacity are contributed by well developed bony thoracic cage, good muscular girth and the respiratory vital capacity. Persons harbouring chronic respiratory diseases, nutritional specially calcium and protein deficiency have sub-standard chest measure.

The recruit should be made to stand erect with his feet together and raise his arms above his chest. The tape should be carefully adjusted round the mid-chest. After the normal chest measure, the candidate is asked to take full breath so as to expand the chest cavity fully. The maximum measure is recorded then. In chronic restrictive long diseases and some cardio-vascular diseases the chest expansion is limited and on forcing, the person gets dyspnoea. At this stage the doctor should look for drooping shoulder, winging of scapular or any abnormal epigastic pulsation which may suggest internal disease.

4. *General Examination*--The doctor should look for anaemia, vericisity of veins, nutritional deficiency, skin diseases, leprotic patches, non-healing ulcer, palpalde lymphnodes, lupus sign,

malar flush, etc. in way of ruling out presence of systemic diseases.

5. The evidence of any hereditary or acquired defect in the body such as bowed legs, knock knee (kissing knee), flat foot, etc. be carefully looked for. Any deformity in the Malleoli or toes which may produce painful condition on wearing heavy ammunition boots for long time, long march or sports activity is to be considered adequate reason for rejection. Shortening or wasting of any limb due to whatever cause are sure cases of unfitness.

6. *The Examination of Eyes*--both for disease and vision in a recruit bears immense importance. The external examination may show presence of any infective eye-disease like conjunctivitis, Keratitis, Corneal ulcer, etc. The accuracy of vision for both near and distant objects must be examined using standard charts to avoid fallacy. Each eye must be examined separately. The defective colour vision must be detected by Ishihara-chart as such defect is sufficient ground for rejection of a candidate. Sufficient allowance must be allowed for posts like followers, clerical and hospital staff but must be strict for driver and fitter service. Any degree of squint is ground for disqualification for fighting force including automobile drivers.

The colour vision defect is almost always since birth and is a defect of permanent nature. The standard of acuity vision may vary with nature of job and age. The recruiting officers may come across such cases while enrolling ex-army personnel.

7. *Adequate Hearing*--capacity is essential for members of police forces. Hearing defect of permanent nature such as nerve deafness if in an candidate, he cannot be recruited to police forces. Although a proper hearing test may not be possible to conduct in the recruitment site, person able to hear 'normal talk' from a twenty feet distance is good enough for police duty.

8. *Good Oral Hygiene*--with healthy sets of teeth and gum is asset for a soldier. The teeth with proper masticating and biting power should be sought for. With this the inspection of

tongue, tonsils and throat should also be completed. Gross defects like hoarseness of voice, defective or stammering speech or gross deviation of nasal septrum must be ruled out.

9. The presence of any big scar on abdomen or renal angle would speak the story of any major surgical procedure the candidate might have undergone in past. Besides, hernia (inguinal or abominal) hydrocele, piles and fissure must be ruled out as such condition would aggravate when the recruit is put to rigorous exercise.

10. *The Respiratory System*– is affected by various pathogenic, environmental and allergic disorders causing chronic illness, detormits, failure of proper growth, reduced tolerance power and worsening in extreme conditions such as cold. This stresses the need for a thorough examination or respiratory system to rule out the possibility of any sort of ailment. In doubtful cases, second opinion by a specialist may be taken and X-ray chest and/or vitalography may be performed before final rejection.

11. *The Cardio-Vascular System* --including blood pressure needs thorough clinical screening before enrollment. The presence of congenital or acquired heart disease may lead to severe limitation in the exercise tolerance and interfere the duties of policemen. Even the functional murmur heard should be properly evaluated. There may be temporary rise of blood pressure due to post exercise and examination fear in the candidates. Such cases must be examined again and again to rule out organic disease. An ECG and specialist opinion should be preferred before hasty rejection.

12. *Neuro-Psychiatric Angle*--The candidate for any post in police force should be free from *Neuro-Psychiatric normal disorders.* Maniac or hysteric symptoms or loss of mental equilibrium are conditions not acceptable in police recruitment. An average intelligence is good enough for constabulary but higher degree of intelligence memory, judgement and mental alertness are required when the candidate is being appointed for post of sub-ordinate officer or directly appointed Gazetted Officers.

As a matter of fact, the recruitment party with limited time and facility is hardly able to conduct all the tests required to judge the suitability of candidates. Because of widespread unemployment the candidates are large in number. Every one of them deserve justice of going through all the tests before they return home. The task of screening of these vast crowd becomes humanly impossible. The medical examination schedule comes only after physical measurement and by then the brighter part of the day is already wasted and the doctor hardly gets natural light to examine the candidates properly. It is only the clinical acumen of the recruiting doctor which plays the major role to determine the standard of screening process. To achieve the best the blue-book instructions are never adequate. There is always a scope to select the best of the lot for this specialised profession.

The enlistment of female constabulary for para-military forces, home-guard or civil police is again a ticklish job. Proper physical standard and medical status are required for police job but for posts in ministerial or hospital cadre, the standards are relaxed. Cases are decided on their own merit. However, any female candidate in any stage of pregnancy can not be appointed to any government post as a general principle. The appointment has to be deferred till delivery or termination. In all such cases the report from a gynaecologist is an integral part of medical examination.

Inspite of the strict recruitment standard, the unattractive salary and perks, the hazardous nature of duties, poor promotional prospect, there have been never any problem of getting adequately suitable candidates to fill up police force vacancies. Rather in many occasions the team finds it difficult to reject some candidate as the vacancies happen to be limited. The large crowd of aspirants on the recruitment days is, undoubtedly, is the effect of population explosion and the resultant high rate of educated unemployed youth in the country.

The Medical Interrogation

Contrary to the popular belief, the personal medical interrogation of police recruits is neither unwanted nor customary. As every government servant has to produce a clean chit in support of his character and antecedents, this procedure is an integral part of recruitment process to bring out any history of illness in past. This is strictly followed in army, the central police organization and some of the state armed police wings. However, the exercise is conveniently avoided in local police enrollments. The armed police forces have their credential in the country for their high standard of discipline and preparedness for duty. A healthy body and a sound mind both are required to attain such state. Hence, medical interrogation is more relevant to armed police situation such as central para-military forces, rapid action force, National Security Guard Commando Service etc. The candidate might have suffered from any disease in the past or a positive family history may be available which may not be detectable at the time of recruitment medical examination. Illness like epilepsy, diabetes mellitus, abdominal tuberculosis familial bleeding disorders, nervous break-down, fainting attack, etc. do not have external clinical evidence to be detected on the spot. Hence, the system of medical interrogation is perfectly in order.

In order to make the exercise of medical interrogation more meaningful the doctor and para-medical staff are required to put sincere efforts to elicit helpful information. The data are likely to be erroneous because of two reasons. Firstly, the candidate may not be able to understand the medical syndrome enquired about and secondly, he may try to hide facts in fear of rejection. Hence, the candidate has to be convinced that the information is just for record and not intended adverse to his/ candidature.

Education and Police Health

The minimum educational qualification for enlistment to constabulary in almost all police forces in India has been made "Tenth class pass". For the follower posts even less education is also permitted. For direct employment to subordinate or Gazetted officer posts, higher qualification like graduation is required. Because of rise in the literacy rate and rising unemployment in the country, the general turn up of candidates is more qualified than required. Hence, the recruited crowd is predominatedly higher educated than required. The trend has helped the men in police force to have concrete concept of better personal hygiene, decent living, seeking immediate medical aid on illness and consciousness towards family planning. Hence, higher education had direct impact on the health of the troops and so enlistment of holders of higher degree/diploma candidates, should be encouraged. But such candidates being over ambitious may easily get frustrated. To avoid such situation, such personnel who are an asset to the force can be offered better incentives. The immediate incentive can be a job incentive by engaging them in scriptory, artistic, or liaison work. The other incentive which can be offered periodically is their selection to higher posts such as sub-inspector, Ministerial Staff, technical posts of signal units to science graduates and using computer educated boys in Data Processing Cell and Criminal Analysis branches through inservice remustering.

Even the elaborate exercise of recruitment with honest purpose of accepting only disease free or fit persons to the police forces may prove fruitless as some silent diseases may be missed, such as diabetes mellitues, myocardia ischaemia or an old healed tuberculosis. Even insisting on the routine investigations may not uncover the underlying disease. No recruitment team can be that perfect to eliminate all ailments. Moreover, human body when subjected to a different environment, food, exercise, etc. is likely to develop illness of any nature.

A police recruit has no typical pattern. Each one of them are drawn from different stock environment and cultural background. His individual peculiarities, food habits and other hobbies and inclinations are sacrificed. He is moulded to lead a close community life under strict disciplinary control, ready to obey order even in hazardous conditions. This meta morphosis from a civilian to a physically, mentally, emotionally and socially fit member of police force is like the way in which with passage of time the transformation of wood to coal and coal to diamond occurs. This involves training and guidance. State of health contributes to standard of fitness and level of devotion to police profession.

Health Education in Police Training

In India, police training centres cater for various groups of police trainees at their entry points and in service advance or orientation programmes. The police forces have three entry levels. The lowermost is at the constabulary level, the middle at Sub-Inspector or Asstt. Sub-inspector level and the upper one for the Officer level. The constabulary which has to undergo a basic training for 36 weeks at the recruits training centre or battalion headquarters follow a well framed schedule and curriculum. The middle level subordinate officers take up similar duration basic course at Police Training College or Central Training Colleges of central para-military forces. These junior officers are practically the 'junior Managers' of the force who work as the links between the superior officers and the constabulary. Finally, there is the upper level entry of directly appointed gazetted officers either of State Police Cadres, Central Police organization cadres of All India Service Cadre like the IPS who come through Service Selection Board or Union Public Service Commission. The IPS officers undergo training in the National Police Academy whereas the State and CPO cadre officers are trained through their own colleges and academies. Administrative, managerial, legal and operational training are supplemented by field exposures and follow up probationership in the Officer Cadres.

Health education is a poorly understood subject. It is mostly confused with medical education and left to be the Doctor's affair. The concept is absolutely wrong. Health education enables the personnel to observe their own health care, get over the false belief and develop power of rational thinking, acquire sound knowledge on health promotion and maintenance and to be health conscious rather than illness phobic for making health their valued asset. Health education sows healthy habits more permanently among the personnel and their families. The invaluable and limitless benefits of health education can not be emphasised more with the limited scope of this book.

Should health education form a part of basic training in police forces? If so why is the matter no longer a proposition? It is an axiom. Hence, needs no discussion. It is agreed in every sphere and forum that health education has a vital role to play and must be included in basic training programme of all police forces. It promotes good personal habits and contributes to achieving positive health morale and well being and reduces vulnerability to diseases. It provides all facilities to live healthily. But only imparting of knowledge brings no relief unless the attitude of the trainee is favourable. The impact effects his family, neighbours and finally the community. But unfortunately such a useful part of training is grossly neglected. The importance of such education is poorly understood by the managers of training programme. Classes ear-marked for health education, first aid, personal hygiene, etc. are conveniently skipped and utilized for other out of curriculum activities. Even in old training institutions proper teaching aids are not available.

The intensive implementation of health education programme is more relevant in the basic training of constabulary since these new recruits are drawn from heterogenous background, have less civil education, poor socio-economic strata and are mostly from rural background. When they are made to lead a police barrack life the practice of personal hygiene principles becomes highly essential. It is one of the mode of manpower development in the police forces. The improvement of standard of living and overall development can be induced through health education. The effect of such education goes a long way in their service career.

The subordinate officers possess higher civil education than the constabulary and the cream is selected for the posts through the competitive examination. These 'middle managers' of police forces manage the crime detection job of police stations or work as platoon commanders in armed police wings, leading operationally pioneer group of trained soldiers. It is expected that they have learnt the basic principles of health keeping. Health education in their training help to acquire better concept of public health matters, sanitary principles followed in barracks, cook houses, water supply, immunization, eradication of fly and mosquitos, etc. They develop better aptitude to a healthy and decent living as a supervisor of troops and they understand the health needs of constabulary under them better. Hence, health education is invaluable to them.

But why should the officers be put through such a rudimentary education system, who are already highly educated and function as senior executives in the police formations. These officers command a larger segment of the force where they also act as planners for over all development of men under their command. This also includes health planning which demands a fair knowledge of public health systems and national and international health regulations. However, their teaching may not be confined to the class rooms. Symposium, guest lectures, demonstration and field visits would be more suitable. Video film show can make better impact. Besides, these senior officers in course of their normal duties, undergo enough mental strain which may lead to develop stress disease in them. Health education would make them conscious about it.

The imparting of health education is relevant to not only police forces, it is also useful to every member of public. Our school text books are poorly designed so far as health education is concerned. The present day popular media like newspapers, radio and television have taken up this task to some extent. Inspite of that, the classical teachings are not unnecessary as the spectrum of study is large enough. The case of sex education which is also a part of health education is worth mentioning. The poor and incomplete knowledge of sex leads to several implications and contacting of diseases. A proper knowledge on the subject helps in character building. But this education is never imparted in schools most probably due to shyness of educators. In police forces, the trainees are grown-up and mature and are under strict disciplinary frame. Sex education can be better given in this stage to boys who would lead 70-80% of their service life in police barracks without family life and prone to extra-marital connection. A fair knowledge would help him prevent sexually transmitted disease, infertility abortions, marital disharmony which may finally end up in divorce or suicides.

To draw a comprehensive course of studies on the health related subjects is purposely avoided in this book. Besides, basic training, there are large number of in-service training, refresher, orientation programmes run by different institutions for all ranks. They range from advance weapon tactics, technical, provisional, administrative or communication matters to counter insurgency and jungle warfare. These forces should also include some classes on relevant health subjects for the benefit of the participants. Some health education topics for inclusion in service courses are suggested.

	Name of Course	*Kind of Health Education suggested*
1.	Administrative Refresher Course for Officers, Commandants and Medical Officers	Stress disorders for such as diabetes, hyper-tension, coronary heart diseases, acid peptic diseases, health planning, national and international health regulations.
2.	Junior Command and Senior Command Course for non Commissioned officers/under officers	Personal hygiene, prevention of malaria and water borne diseases, family planning methods, prevention of venereal diseases, AIDS, hepatitis, adverse drug reactions and self doctoring.
3.	Senior Inspector, Refresher Course	Recognition and management of old age health problems, epidemic control and notifiable diseases.
4.	Motor Transport Officers and Quarter Master Course	First aid on accidental injuries, field management fractures, bleeding, transportation of injured, management of accidental poisoning by chemicals.

5.	Tear Smoke Course	Prevention and treatment of accidental MIC intoxication, artificial respiration.
6.	Weapon Tactic Course	Field management of bullet injury, control of haemorrhage.
7.	Jungle Warfare Course	First aid in snake bite, Scorpion and insect bite. Field dressing procedures, water discipline.
8.	Map Reading and Shooting Courses	Care of eye, regular check up and treatment of eye, Field first aid of bullet injury and haemorrhage.
9.	Unarmed Combat Course	Knowledge of muscular system. Management of sprain and pulls physio-therapy and Infra-red Ray Treatment.
10.	Bugler's course	Respiratory problems and their field management, tuberculosis.
11.	For Cooks and *Safai Karmacharies*, Barbers,	Personal hygiene, water borne disease, food poisoning, Intestinal parasites, tuberculosis, inspection of eatables such as fruits, vegetables, eggs, meat, fish and chicken, skin diseases.
12.	Fire Fighting Course	First aid for burn, artificial respiration, rescue and relief operations, care for survivor of drowning accident.
13.	Medical Officers Basic Course	Statistical and economical topics on population explosion, family

		planning. Epidemic control, theories and practice, sports medicine, development of teaching aids for various courses in police forces. Hospital Management.
14.	Medical officers Refresher Course	Advanced training in disaster management, Laparoscopic family planning operations, recent advances in Medical Sciences, modern diagnostic and therapeutic procedures. Hospital Administration.
15.	Hospital Staff Basic Course	All first aid and nursing procedures, Laboratory and CT techniques, hygiene, sanitation, epidemic control, drug regulation, management of ADR, Cardio-respiratory emergencies.

Thus, health education and first aid training should be an integral part of every police training programme. Every trained police man in the country should be a trained. First Aid Worker also capable of helping his colleagues or neighbour in hours of need, in addition to shaping his own personal life style as an ideal citizen. We are all familiar with the old proverbial saying 'Every policeman is a citizen with uniform and every citizen is a policeman without uniform. The upholders of police philosophy would rewrite the old saying as-'Every policeman is also a trained first aid worker and health educator and an exemplary citizen with best form of personal hygiene'.

5

Impact of Police Duty on Health

Police duty is not a job, it is a profession, like any other profession and a person who joins a police service, enters the profession. And once a man is in this profession, he is there almost permanently. The degree ot devotion and professionalism required to be a member in any other profession is also required for this profession. One who enters the police force, almost denounces the rest of the world. For him, his own duty and the honour and dignity of the Khaki-clad profession comes first than any other thing. The sacrifice is unlimited and at times the policeman has to sacrifice the comfort, life and safety of his own, of his family and dependents, friends and relatives without even waiting for what the government or the society gives him in return or how his action is evaluated.

The thinkers of Occupational Medicine wonder whether like any other occupation, the police work has any relevant impact on the health of the policeman. Considering the working environment in which the police or the armed police force have to work, the stress and strain received, it creates genuine doubt in one's mind that there must have been some impact or the other. The olden day police force bear the image of healthy strongmen on the streets or check-gate. But over the decades, the nature of police duties has changed in magnitude. The change has been necessitated due to change in the pattern of law and order, more so to that of pre-Independent India. The irruption of separatist and emotional groups in different parts of the country has required the rapid expansion of the existing police forces, imparting of special and advance trainings, creation of specialised groups among them, opening of woman para-military force, Rapid Action Force, etc. have changed the face of police entirely. Besides, the rapid movements to the *"hot spots"* have been the corner stone of armed police duty.

There have been several factors which have direct impact on the health of a policeman on duty. Let us now consider some of the factors.

1. General Factors

Barring a few civil police posts, the police life is largely "Barrack Life". The armed police force personnel soon after the recruitment, start living in police campuses, in specially designed police barracks meant for singlemen. These barracks with long halls and broad corridors and lobbies cater for large number of men who join training and after training duties, short courses, refresher classes, etc. These barracks, although some of them have modern facilities of sanitation, are over crowded and have ill ventilation. Due to rapid expansion, some facilities are not made available to all men and one has to be content with canvas accommodation, of tent with open bench latrine and water supply through tankers. The young trainee recruits who are still to recover from the home-sickness completely, lose their old social contacts. In the new locations also, their movements outside the camp is very much restricted. The separation from family members, friends and relatives bring the initial set back in mind which they are made to forget with busy training programmes, hard to digest lessons, jungle training, long marches, range firing, sports and games, barrack maintenance and other activities. The sharing of food from the common kitchen offers him no choice to food. His likings and dislikings are sacrificed. The effect of climate of training centre also plays vital role in case the same is situated far away from his home town. The language difficulty, particularly among the South Indian boys also makes them feel out of place till they learn the training language or local language. In the Central para-military forces the language of training is '*Roman Hindi*' (Language of Hindi written in English script) and Hindi. Although, there is a system of teaching Hindi to non-Hindi speaking recruits, adequate knowledge of the new language cannot be imparted so quickly. Besides, the teachers also teach in Hindi medium. Hence, the system is not totally successful. In the state police forces, the recruits and instructors are mostly local and conversant with local language. So whatever may be the medium of training, the explanations are elaborated in the local language. Hence, such difficulties are easily over-come.

The initial basic training of new police recruits is known for its rigorous nature. The training includes regimentation to uniformed service and endurance to the hard police life. The recruits who are non-serious to their police life and with no determination are lacking devotion, find their way out of the career. Many boys find their solace through the hospital services by exaggerating their minor illnesses. Some find respite by pleasing their immediate seniors by some other means. A few of them leave for home on short casual leave but never return to the khaki life and finally give up the job.

2. The Exposures and Associations

When the trained policeman enters to active duty phase, he is exposed to the world of crime, lawlessness, investigation, court proceedings, punishments, etc., as a member of civil police. In the armed wings, the policeman comes across crowd control, border patrolling, guarding vital installations, VIP security, anti-terrorist police action, etc. All these are a complete diversion from the normal civil life. In the society, the policeman is regarded as a guardian of peace and harbinger of communal amity. But he is also looked differently, as an agency of the ruling political and administrative set up and hence, he is not believed. The civilians are hardly civil to them.

During the course of his police career, he is exposed to the under-world of criminals, provocation to bribery, alcoholism and other forms of bad habits. Strict, honest and rigid police officers and constabulary who do not fall so easily in their trap are threatened for life, kidnapping of their children, etc. The nature of duty is odd and mentally/physically exhaustive. The dealing with gamblers, smugglers, black marketeers is full of risk. The operations like raids, searches, ambush, follow-ups, criminal investigations and in other similar practices there is no fixed hours of duty. Hence, the policeman has to sacrifice his own comforts and remains tense and alert. This increases the stress and strain in the body and mind of the policemen. There is no proper timing for lunch or dinner and the troops have to move on very short notice without even time for any preparation. Frequent movements in armed forces bring sudden radical change in climate which affects their health adversely. These factors like undue stress and strain, irregularities in food timing, long hours of duty, sudden movements, etc. contribute heavily in deterioration of the health standard of police force.

As the para-military forces serve as the second line of defence and border patrolling is part of their legitimate duties, the members of these forces are exposed to international conflicts at the frontiers and sustain bullet injuries from the enemy forces. In such situations, the troops hardly get a chance to proceed on their annual earned leave and remain cut off from their families. Being unable to attend to their personal social and property problems, they remain worried and tense. The police force is also the target of anti-social elements in insurgent areas and the unlawful crowd on the streets against whom they have to raise their arms as a part of their *bona-fide* duty. These crowds and extremists are members of the same society to which the armed police personnel belong. They have also social obligations towards them but for their nature of duty. This dual action of policeman in disturbed operational areas is unique and has an adverse impact on their psyche.

3. Mental Pressures

The pressure on the mind of a policeman on duty is tremendous. As already elaborated, the job assigned to him is of an awesome nature and hence, as a human being the policeman has to perform the same with hesitation and against his will and conscience. He first tries to avoid and bypass it. But after motivation, he is compelled to do it. The senior officers have to exert their administrative authority and tactics to get the work done from the constabulary. The reason of initial reluctance is also obvious. The police action being directly against the criminals and notorious persons, the police force is in constant threat from these bad elements. They try to overcome the police action by bribery, intimidation and other illegal means. The situation becomes still complicated when any of their friends or relatives are involved in criminal cases when the investigating policemen has to exhibit his extra-ordinary devotion to duty. Such psychological trauma may well bring any degree of mental breakdown in the policeman.

Working under constant pressure from various sources the policeman on duty has to adopt a balanced policy in mind guided by his personal attitude, conscience, family background and his overall mental capability. Mostly, his own inner feelings are sacrificed at the alter of duty but all such pressures leave irrepairable damaging effect on the body and mind of the policeman, finally, manifesting in the form of diseases. Conditions like hyper-tension, Acid-peptic diseases, diabetes mellitus and a host of other diseases are common in police occupation. A group of them with a type personality of an over enthusiastic worker suffer mostly from coronary heart disease and mental breakdown. This brings an abrupt fall on the pitch of activities of police force. To overcome the pressure on mind, the policemen seek constant assistance from the medical men for better sleep, relaxation and energy yielding capacity through drugs. Some adopt to alcoholism for mental relaxation, which again is addictive and the cause of permanent organic damage to the body. Unable to give up the habit, men suffer from mal-nutritions, cirshosis of liver and cardio-myopathies. The family suffers due to loss of money or death of bread earner, with long standing effect on their future lives.

4. Internal Factors

In addition to the various external pressure on the policeman on duty, there are large number of internal factors which also contribute heavily to design his life and career. The spectrum of this is wide. To start with, we find that the work-load is quite heavy. The over-duty throughout the year has constant deteriorating effect on the health. Other factors like financial hardship with meagre salary to meet the challenge of high cost of living and to meet the social obligations play vital role for his mental freedom to perform duty. This provokes him to be dishonest and accept illegal gratification in cash or kind. Lack of incentive in the job and failure to receive recognition and reward for good work retards his police dynamism. The failing health status of self and family keeps him physically unprepared and mentally occupied. Old age sluggishness also hampers the police duty. Finally, the monotony of police duty renders him useless for a real police job except that of routine nature.

The above account has been only a cross sectional analysis of the visible factors affecting the health of a policeman on active duty. There have been a vast world of invisible factors which are strictly personal, familial and peculiar to the particular individual which have never come to light. There has been no systematic or investigative research on the subject. A thorough critical analysis of the factors leading to physical and mental ailments of armed police forces can no doubt discover interesting facts. The single major factor "Stress" needs further elaboration.

Role of Stress

As already described in previous paragraphs, stress is the most common single disease producing factors in the policeman on active duty. But stress itself is not a disease. It is the "Stimulus-response-complex" All stress are not harmful. A physical or psychological stress may even promote the resistance phenomena. It is initially beneficial when applied in tolerable degree and spread over a reasonably tolerable period. The biological stress is caused by infection, physical stress by factors like extreme heat, cold, burn, injury; where as the psychological stress is produced by lack of congenial atmosphere at home, office, neighbourhood, clubs, relations, proximity to aggressive or irritative personality or social change. The body has its own protective mechanism in stressful situations which is called "General Adaptation" in which the pituitary adrenal-axis plays the vital role. The failure of adaptation because of over-dose of stress or prolonged period leads to "Stage of Exhaustion" or imbalance between Attack and Defence Mechanism. Such imbalance or mal-adaptation leads to development of "Stress Diseases".

The stress diseases are becoming more prevalent in armed forces. This group of diseases is also common in general public in higher economic strata, modernised well-to-do, professionals and bussiness classes. The group includes a large spectrum of disease entities of diverse nature such as Psychological disorders, Hyper-tension, Nephroselerosis, Collagen diseases, some skin conditions, Ischaemic and other athero-sclerotic heart diseases, Acid-peptic diseases of stomach and intestine, thyrotoxieosis, etc. With advancement of modern diagnostic and clinical procedures, more and more stress disorders are being added to the list. It is also clarified that stress alone may not be single contributor of any of the disease process unless the other causative factors are also present. More correctly it can be a precipitating factor of a disease of multiple aetiology. Factors like vulnerable personality, environmental influence, cultural pattern, habit and behaviour pattern of the individual and degree of resistance to stress play pivotal role.

Modern civilization with its accelerated tempo of life has definite impact on the human psyche to start a chain of reactions, although the target organ is determined by genetic and constitutional factors, and not always the mind as popularly believed. The incidence of stress diseases is in rising trend in all the three wings of armed forces, army, navy and air-force. The incidence among officers is nearly three times higher than that of "all rank" incidence. This group is tending to dominate the morbidity pattern in forces. Although the statistical data for police forces are not available, the pattern is presumably not of any diverse nature from the regular army pattern. About 20% of total manpower wastage is caused by invalidation and death can be attributed to this group directly or indirectly.

The medical scientists and administrators who are at the helm of affairs of police forces are invited to focus their research to identify cases, arrange complete analysis, collection of data and evolve eradication and preventive measures of stress disease. A few measures are suggested as follows :

1. Careful selection of recruits so as to avoid entry of undesirable persons in police forces.
2. Creation of healthy and congenial environment during the budding stages like basic training and initial years of service.
3. Proper motivation for police life, help development of aptitude towards camp life, separated life, exposure to criminal and terrorist environment.
4. Identification of deserving cases for incentive and create opportunity to rise rather than "rotting" with less deserving persons. The facility for career promotion and to show his extra capability, merit or talent, must be created.
5. Proper guidance to improve in the line of his aptitude, to promote his physical and mental health, to ensure congenial atmosphere in working place and cordial relationship among fellow-mates.
6. Prompt payment of dues, sanction of loans and advances to overcome economic constraint, timely promotion and other service benefits must be ensured.
7. Grant of adequate quantum of leave and leave travel benefits to meet his social and familial circle, opportunity to relax and change in environment etc.
8. Moral building should be encouraged through proper education, training, motivation, etc.
9. Early recognisation and weeding out of vulnerable personalities of stress diseases or maladaptation

cases. There is no quantitative test for identification of these cases, close observations and careful questioning may help to give indication.

10. Proper man-management is the key factor of controlling the rising menace in police forces.

In the present day police forces, the most difficult problem in management is to motivate the constabulary to do the monotonous repetitive nature of job although, not hard to perform. Besides, the lack of aptitude and dislike to a particular job lead them to feign sickness and avoid such duties. Now with the incoming of large crowd of educated youth to the police forces, the job of "officers' orderly" in which the constable has to look into the personal work of his superior officer is not liked. The National Police Commission set up in 1977 has recommended for abolition of the system from the police forces which has been followed very promptly. These constabulary engaged in orderly job were also vigilant for purpose of safety and security of the officer, his family members, attending telephone calls and helping officer to prepare for regimental duties. To cover these aspects of the system, a new "Security Aid" system has been started by the All India Forces and some State Reserve Police Forces. Many such experiments are on trial, as part of the over-hauling reform of the police system in the country.

Inspite of the fact that the nature of job has been modified, there is general dislike for the job from the active service population of the troops. It is overcome by lots of motivation, allurement for fringe benefits and personal comforts. Men, generally, after the age of 50 years, who normally do not fit to the hectic police duties are volunteers for the job. Some State police organisations have adopted a novel system to solve the problem. They made a separate cadre of "Fellow to Officer" in the follower grade of pay. The men recruited against such posts are meant for the duties similar to security aids in CPOs. This also helps in saving the active duty trained man-power from such unpleasant job and reduce dissatisfaction in the troops.

Consequences of Policeman in Tension

Before concluding this chapter, a detailed account of the grave consequences of the policeman in tension would not be out of place. A policeman who is responsible for public peace and relief of social tension, at times remains in tension. A tense policeman develops disease leading to chronic illness. His illness not only affects his own efficiency in work but his family also suffers financially. The illness is worsened by poor nutrition in diet. His work output drastically falls. Factors like over duty, frustration, lack of incentive or reward for good work further brings down the work output and efficiency of the policeman. If the police force suffers from such setback, it becomes ineffective for any special duty for which they are meant. The ineffective police force becomes unable to control any law and order situation or any other duty assigned to it. This being the active arm of the ruling government, lawlessness and chaos prevails throughout the country, finally, posing threat to the democratic set-up. Hence, the tension or the ill health of a single policeman is never an isolated event. It has the relevance to the entire democratic set-up of the country. Such cases cannot be neglected. In the greater interest of the country, the relief of tension and full treatment of his illness is essential. Any left over tension, dissatisfaction, grievance or illness is likely to rise again and again like a fire not extinguished fully.

6

The Doctors and the Health Set-up

Health, like happiness is more of an abstract term for subjective consideration rather than for objective quantification. It is the description of a relative condition of a person representing the degree of his effectiveness in particular circumstances in his hereditary, physical and cultural environment. Medicine, is the art of applying the best of all sciences known to the mankind for his benefit. Physicians through the ages have embraced all the bio-scientific, technological and therapeutic advances to meet the challenge of patient care and let the profession to survive in the passage of time and emerge as the inseparable factor for the evolution of human race.

The science of healing is in practice since pre-historic times in some form or other. People who were ill were looked after by their families and relatives for many centuries. With the advent of concept like isolation, prevention, nursing care, early cure to prevent personal and economic pressure of illness and to give comfort to the patient, the systematic institutional care came into existence. The delivery of health care services through hospitals (derived from the word Hospitality) gained momentum with the incoming of surgery, Maternity-child care activities, Laboratory, X-ray, etc. Industrialisation, education and health consciousness increased the demand of these services many fold, even the professionalism leading to commercialisation.

India, receiving its dose of western civilization has broadly accepted the modern medicine system as the major determinant in its health care culture. The mushrooming of hospitals, medical colleges and ancillary institutions specially after Independence in public and private sectors have revolutionised the field of health care. With 128 medical colleges and around 34000 hospitals in the country the strength of hospital beds is around 6.5 lakhs in a country with 88 crore population. Though the medical colleges have annual admission capacity of 15000 for basic doctors like MBBS, only 3.75 lakhs doctors are available to serve the teaming millions. Only one physician is available in a population of 3700 which is grossly inadequate in comparison to the developed countries. The matter further worsens with tendency of qualified doctors prefering urban practice rather than to go to the remote corners of the country.

But, is it not tantalising to hear that we have more policemen in the country than medical-men. The figures of 1984 states that all the State police forces in the country including their armed wings accumulated together counts 7.8 lakhs. To add to this, the five major para-military Central forces (BSF, CRPF, ITBP, CISF, RPF) constitute a total of 4.24 lakhs. Even after over-looking the sizable number of non-uniformed policemen, the smaller forces, home-Guards, RAW and other investigating agencies, one policeman is available per 600 civilians. (All figures are rounded off). The cancerous growth in the size of police forces both in State and Central level holds the barometer of the criminality and lawless environment of the country.

The other side of the story is also interesting. The policemen in course of discharging their *bona-fide* duties succumb to the situation. Literally, they are fighting continuously an "*Undeclared War*". The National Crime Record Bureau (MHA) records show that in the last 35 years (1954-1989), 1,10,173 policemen were injured and 6598 have laid their lives while on duty. In other words, on an every year average 3148 persons are being injured (8.6 persons daily) and 188 persons are being killed (one life every two days). This heavy toll of trained manpower is a collossal loss to the country's economy, damaging to the police moral and encouraging to the destructive and secessionist forces. The shocking tale of police casuality, justifies the formation of specialised and inbuilt medical wings in every police organisation.

Health and fitness are part of police life and hence, doctors, hospitals and drugs are the constant accompaniments. In the State police setup, every district police HQ, armed police camps and training centres are provided with medical cover, normally drawing their staffing and budgeting from the Health Department of the State Government. Such arrangement was also the usual practice in many para-military police forces upto late sixties and early seventies. But subsequently, the forces have reorganised their set-up on a need-based manner. The forces have to equip themselves with highly sophisticated weaponary, advanced training and skilled weapon tactices. With the changing pattern of law and order and border situation, the age old system of "borrowed" medical service with civilian doctors and para-medical staff did not fit the system. The history of para-military forces in India in the sixth and seventh decade of the century saw the creation of para-military police medical cadres in the line of Army Medical Corp (AMC). The State police forces with limited or no movements, however, still continue with the medical cover provided from State Medical Cadre. The local State Government hospitals and the medical college hospitals are pressed into service in hours of need.

The Central para-military forces (Central Police Organisations) came to existence mostly in post-independent era except the Assam Rifles and the Central Reserve Police Force. The CRPF traces back its origin in late thirties and rejuvinated under the blessings of Sardar Vallabhbhai Patel (The first Home Minister of Independent India). These forces have undergone thorough reform, re-organisation and need-based development. The nucleus of medical element in each force were formed with deputationist from Central Health Service (CHS) doctors, but soon crystallised to fully developed medical cadre of their own under patronage of Ministry of Home Affairs, Government of India. The evolutionary changes that have undergone are marked with homogenisation by combatisation and rank structure. The service conditions in these cadres still follows the pay parity with the CHS doctors. The Central Industrial Security Force (CISF) because of its wide spread deployment and contact, chiefly with the industrial establishments, has not felt the need of creating an elaborate health care coverage and has limited its service to isolated pockets like training centres and administrative establishments. For the rest of the force, they are dependent on the services of medical section of the industrial unit they are protecting. Employees State Insurance Scheme (ESIS) has their own chain of hospitals and medical aid centres which cater to the needs of the industrial workers as well as the CISF men. The Assam Rifle enjoys the distinction of being the oldest para-military force in the country with a history of around 160 years. The force has its deployment mostly in the North Eastern India, has permanent contonments and are less mobile in nature. It has a close unbilical link with the Indian Army and the medical set up is run as a joint enterprise of civilian and AMC doctors. The Border Security Force (BSF), the Central Reserve Police Force (CRPF) and Indo-Tibetan Border Police (ITBP) have their established cadre of medical and para-medical staff with large chain of hospitals throughout the country.

Looking at the vastness of the country, the deteriorating trend of law and order, the vigilant patrolling of the extensive land and sea borders and the growing insurgency and militancy in different parts of the country, has become the order of the day. The need of a competent medical service which can march in a parallel column with the advancing force was the hard felt need. The traditional and dependent arrangement with the local hospitals had outlived its utility. Of course, it is no axaggeration to say that all those civil and military medical establishments have gladly extended their services to the police forces actively involved at the scene of riot, rally,. election, natural calamity under tense situation. The policeman deserves the best form of treatment and nursing care in own force hospitals to reduce loss of police man-days and to avoid security hazard to them. Hence, the dealing of the police force patients has grown into a speciality with knowledge of associated rules and procedures. This virtually demanded the Government of India, through the Ministry of Home Affairs, to decide setting up of a chain of Central Police Organisation (CPO) hospitals in different parts of the country. The location of hospitals, their size, command and control, management and budgeting has been ear-marked. This scheme in its fully grown form, is expected to be a remarkable success and usher a new era in the field of police medical service in the country. The combatisation of doctors and para-medical staff has brought the new wave of discipline, smartness, regimentation and dutifulness.

The traditional police doctors of the past, bear the image of having engaged in the various forensic medical activities dealing with criminals for injury, postmortem, victims of rape, murder, criminal abortions, etc. helping the police and court in investigation and legal proceedings. But, the present day members of police medical service, are devoted mostly in clinical and administrative work in a changed concept of police medical service. The police force hospital play a vital social and regimental roles in a way the other hospitals would not have been able to do. A few of them are listed below :

1. Medical documentation of all important medical, prophylaxis and personal events in the career of a police force jawan, aiming to keep him physically fit and mentally alert all the time.

2. Detection and prompt treatment of any concealed disease which the patient may be ignorant of.

3. Prevention of self doctoring by the members of police force by making medical facilities available in close proximity.

4. The affairs of health of a policeman should be in the full knowledge of his doctor (authorised medical attendant)

and his unit's commanding officer, and with their close collaboration the policeman gets full benefit for treatment of any disease or injury which is directly attributable to the nature of his duty. On the event of accidental injury, loss of any limb or sense organ, or death, the loss is adequately compensated and his dependents are granted with pensionary benefits as per rules.

5. On the event of any disease or injury which may be aggravated by continuous rigorous duty or exercise, the man gets rest or excuse from duty on the recommendation of doctor.
6. After the clinical cure, from an infective disease, the person can be kept in isolation for the purpose of quarantine on the advise of doctor. Otherwise, such person can be a potential source of spread of the disease in the police community.
7. Periodic inspection of special category staff such as food handlers, mess boys, water carriers, *Safai Karamcnaris* help in detection of carrier state of parasitic and gastro-intestinal diseases and thereby saving the police camp from the fury of epidemics.
8. Maintenance of ideal sanitary state in barracks and cook houses, control of epidemics, control of mosquito and fly menace, dog nuisance, etc. Prophylaxis measures such as inoculation and vaccination, etc. and motivation for family planning operation to eligible couple are also done.
9. To identify and deal officially with any case of malingerer who feign illness to avoid duties of hard nature.
10. To prevent police personnel from contacting civil population, frequently, which may lead to leakage of operational secrecy thereby avoid sabotage by destructive anti-social elements.

This is only a brief summary of regimental roles of police force hospitals. This book devotes a separate chapter for detail account of the role and responsibilities of such hospitals. It will not be out of place to say that the activities of police force hospitals have been highly appreciated by the society, the press, the political and medical dignitaries and intelligentia of the country. Maintenance and upkeeping of the standard of the hospitals have been exemplary.

The Doctors

The association of a medical set-up with the armed police organisation speaks of the happy story of men of arms and men of medicine, marching hand in hand in war and peace. The emotional attachment of both the communities is age old in army formations. War are lost and won based on health and moral of the troops. The patient-doctor relationship has been a way of life and doctors are respected in the force as friend, philosopher and guide. The role of doctors in the police forces can be summarised with the following words, although they do not limit their role in any field.

1. **The Healer.** The clinical duties of medical men come as the foremost one and establish their basic professional credential. The security forces and their families draw their medical attendance from their own force doctors for all practical purposes except when such coverage is not available. In all such cases, they have to depend on civil hospitals or nearby force hospitals.

2. **The Guide.** The police force hospitals are organised in need based fashion. Hence, many uncommon investigations and special treatment facilities are not available. As a result a large number of patients have to be referred to nearby medical college, district hospital, private clinics or laboratory etc. As a layman, the patient is not aware of where he should persue his further treatment. In suchcases, the doctors of police force hospitals serve as guide where the patients can get best treatment for his nature of ailment and other requirements.

3. **The Educator.** The doctor's role as health educator to the troops, families and community is appreciable. The general public of the camp consisting of the force members and their dependants are drawn from various parts of the country, remote

villages and from all socio-economic groups. The knowledge of health education such as child care, decent living, family planning, personal hygiene, nutrition etc are imparted regularly through consultation, exhibition, lecture and organisation of camp periodically. First-aid training is given to recruits and drivers. All these activities help improve the quality of life.

4. **The Counsellor.** Medical counselling is one of the ill undustood subject in our society. The counselling is done by experts through study of cases, analysis of investigation reports and contact with patient and their relatives. The complicated problems of hereditary and genetic diseases, familial bleeding disorders, disposal of malformed toctus, unwanted pregnancies, sexual disharmony, marriage of genetic carriers of genetic and familial diseases and a host of other cases are solved. It is beneficial to the family as well as to the society.

5. **The Moral Booster.** The very presence of doctors in the vicinity of police force lines keeps the moral of the troops in high profile. The pre-induction motivation in insurgency areas is best done by doctors by reassurance and keeping them fit physically and mentally. The families on the base camps are well looked after by the force doctors providing mental relief for troops to fight in advanced frontiers. Doctors and hospital staff are the chief consolators to an ailing policeman.

6. **The Public Health Consultant.** The medical officer in-charge of the police force hospital is the authority to advise the administrative officers on the matters of hygiene and sanitations, epidemic prevention and control, ideal drinking water supply, disposal of wastes and all other public health matters. The periodic inspection of camp areas, food handlers, ration supply items, dry, fresh and non-vegetarian cooking and eating places helps in prevention of various communicable diseases. He is also concerned about environmental measures, fly and mosquito control, stray dog control etc. In the duty battalion, the doctor's services are the best form of welfare measure the unit can provide to the men. The advice of rest on medical ground by doctor is the respile for men from the hazardous duty environment and a quarantine measure.

7. **The Collaborator.** The medical men by virtue of their profession are approachable by all sections of people. They establish the vital link between the public and the administrators of police force. Besides some medico-administrative problems, such as medico-legal cases, malingerers, psychopaths, drug addicts, alcoholics, pathological gamblers do occur in police force lines. Such problems are solved by close collaboration of medical and administrative executives.

8. **The Philanthropist.** The doctors of the force serve as the active philanthropists because of their organisational and participation skill in relief and rescue operations, in accidents, natural calamities, fire, riot etc. Their actions are not only to benefit the members of the force but civilian public also. The organisation of blood donation camp for needy patients, child health camp, immunisation camp,eyedonation camp, cataract operation camp, nutritional survey, midday-meal programme in schools and regular medical general check-up camps are some of their laudable performances. Some battalions and establishments of police forces adopt a village for the all round development of the village including education, employment, health, sanitation, drinking water, nutrition, childcare etc. The doctors play a major role in such programmes.

Even with large number of qualified specialists of various disciplines available in the para-military forces, the medical set-up do not seem to be fully organised, in matters of hospital planning and man-power planning. It has several lacuna which need rectification. So far, the hospital's locations have been decided as per the concentration of the troops. It is a well known fact that small hospitals cannot cater to all special services. Some basic disciplines have to be common to all. Further, each hospital should be designed, staffed and equipped to provide one or more advance speciality service. The placement of expert hands is not so rationalised although all the Base Hospitals have been rendering best speciality services, drawing maximum patients from all parts of the country. The meticulous planning can substantially reduce the dependance on the advanced medical centres or medical colleges hospitals outside force. Inspite of the remarkable improvement since their formation, the growth and development of the hospitals have been evolutionary, need based and visibly slow. The administrative and official bottle-necks are chiefly responsible for this. One single argument which is almost always brought in favour of the baseline medical service in police forces is that the medical set-up deals with basically a healthy population. But the logic is not so tenable. Although the high health profile of troops is an aggreable preamble, it does not cover a large part of the story. The dependants who also form a major part of the beneficiaries need the service more than the fighting policemen. Men who left their families for long time in their native places, where treatment facilities are not available or in case available, is very expensive, arrange treatment of their dependants in the medical centres of police force. Over the decades the dependants have contributed substantially towards bed occupancy, OPD attendance, dispensary expenditure, use of health transport and other ancillary services of hospitals. The acceptors of family planning methods have been most frequent visitors to the hospitals. Policemen on active duty hesitate to undergo family planning operation in fear of subsequent adverse effects on their working capacity. Hence, in force hospitals tubectomy out numbers vasectomy.

In the planning and organisational set up of any department or ministry other than the Health Ministry itself, the doctors and medical branch enjoy a backseat, away from the mainstream of activities and treated as a "Service Group", rather than a technical or professional support to the department. The reasons for this may be best known to the brass board office Bosses of such organisation. Any conservative evaluation may blame the age old rivalry between the technocrat and bureaucrats. The problem does not look to be simple and superficial. The malady is deep rooted. Inspite of adopting the century old army model of medical service in the police forces, the cadres have failed to attract the best medical talents in the country. After delinking from the Ministry of Health, the Central Police Organisations are running their own cadre since the early seventies. The forces have never been able to fill up all the posts with increasing number of vacancies. The matter has been examined in several government and non-government forums. Some of the common facts which have been repeatedly brought out are discussed below.

1. Although these cadres would have worked more efficiently in a compact set up under the disciplinary frame-work of police forces, the lack of meticulous planning and organisation has left the cadre in shambles. Hence, the posts can hardly give any assurance on the fate of qualified doctors who are just out of the academic atmosphere of medical institutions.

2. The cancerous growth of the forces in the last two decades have increased the work-load manifold at the grassroot level but expansion of facilities, staff and infrastructure have been unaffected. The existing facilities have been sized away rendering the same to be ineffective one, Hence, widespread adhocism prevails.

3. The monotony of police life and isolation of duty battalion in the field areas are also matters of dislinking to the young ambitious medical graduates. Frequent movements of troops with uncertainty of situation, poor state of accommodation and lack of other basic amenities are repelling factors for young medical-men.

4. So long as the doctor is a bachelor he tolerates all such difficulties of a duty battalion. But once he starts a family his problems are multiplied. In the duty battalions nobody is allowed to keep their family with them because of nature of duty, frequent movements and the poor state of accomodation. This upsets the family life and subsequently the children's education suffer the most. Doctors who have the sole responsibility of looking after their old parents and other dependants, cannot persue the job in police forces. They prefer to do away with the para-military job and join any civil or private job even with lesser emoluments, compensating the loss through private practice.

5. The pay scales of CPO doctors are adopted in toto from CHS. Most of the state governments have also equalised

the pay scales of doctors with that of their Central counterparts. Besides in state government jobs private practice in spare time is allowed. Hence, the Central Health Service and the Police (CPO) jobs are no longer alluring, the latter receiving last priority.

6. The CPO doctors are combatised for limited purposes, for duty, discipline and conduct. The rank and badges authorised to doctors does not entitle them to the equal pay-scales with their police counterparts. Being combatised, they undergo all the rigors of force life but benefits and privileges are denied to them. This is the pinch felt by them white apron clad professionals, who have virtually turned to khaki wearing police doctors.

7. The promotional prospects in the cadres is minimal as compared to CHS or General duty police officers of the force. The rapid expansion of the force increases posts at the lowest grade but does not automatically increase the posts at higher grades. Hence, any expansion of the forces bring extra work-load but does not improve scope in the career. Hence, those who join service by compulsion, or in ignorance of the situation, get frustrated and prepare for premature departure searching for greener pastures.

8. The scope of higher study of doctors reduces drasticaly, after joining a job in any CPO. It is because of lack of facilities for preparation for the competitive entrance examinations, frequent change of postal address, delayed mail service in far flung places, delayed or no delivery of national newspapers in remote localities berefts them of watching advertisements and admission notices, non-availability of study leave before at least five years of service and so on. Further, if at all selected for any P.G. Course by own efforts or sponsored by the force, the three year post P.G. liability service bond blocks prospects. These factors dissuade the ambitious doctors to continue in service. To enter into P.G. study in any medical disciplines is a rare opportunity in these days of

competition, and no doctor would like to forego such a chance. Hence, doctors prefer to give up this job and join higher study.

9. Execution of bond is again a negative factor. Some central police forces execute bond with the new entrant doctors to serve a minimum period failing which they are penalised heavy cash payment, although no extra benefit is granted to them in service. Such arrangement compels him to serve knowling his future plight fully well.

10. The CPO medical cadres have some posts of doctors in far-flung places, hill stations, snow-bound areas and other interrior frontiers with unfavorable climatic condition and communication facilities. Such postings are not acceptable to the doctors from health and social point of view.

11. Long transfers from one end of the country to another, is another hallmark of CPO service. The officer has to move with his family and household goods against all adverses like long journey, change of climate, language and environment. He incurs heavy expenditures on the transport of personal goods. Such changes affect hobbies like gardening, clublife, social contact, official contact, loss of contact from relatives, friends etc. Search for good match for marriagable children suffers set back affecting social life. Effects of multiple language deforms the purity and fluency of mother tongue. They are unable to attend on the needs of family specially on the illness, death of parents, birth of children etc. The doctors who value these social events higher than their job reject the central para-military jobs.

12. Inability to join professional learned bodies like Indian Medical Association, Association of Physicians and other speciality associations, for developing professional brotherhood and continue learning through their academic activities. Such facilities are not available in remote areas and disruption due to frequent movements, cost them heavily as far as a normal life is concerned.

The CPO medical cadres with all their draw-backs and limitations have the charm of social safety, clublife, Mess facilities for bachelors and force bachelor officers medical facilities are one of the best in the country. The pay and emoluments being at par with the CHS counterparts, the doctors of CPOs have not much valid reason to be unhappy. Other service conditions are almost the inseparable part of police force life and hence acceptability should improve. The Government is considerate about the hardship the doctors are facing in the para-military forces and more and more benefits are expected to be in the pipeline.

The Para-Medical Staff

The medical cadre of armed police forces not only include the qualified doctors but they run the show with the positive assistance of a large army of para-medical and semi-skilled workers. The para-medicals such as the pharmacists, laboratary technicians, radiographers, staff nurses, dieticians, Matrons, ECG operators, Ultra-sonographer, Physio-therapists etc. from the main bulk of workers in various sections and sub-sections of the hospitals. Besides they are also managing the M.I. Rooms set up at the duty battalions, detachment camps, jungle camps, firing ranges, sport meets, fairs and festivals, accident and natural calamities relief teams, recruitment parties, and so on. Their services are available day and night to the police forces carrying out the dare devil operations against terrorists and anti-social elements. The other associated "hospital assistants" include the ward boys, ward girls, nursing assistants, operation theatre assistant, *ayas*, rece ptionist, registration clerk, and storeman etc. The work in hospital is round the clock. Hence, a continuous duty roster has to be maintained caring for the ailing police community and their dependants. These staffs virtually maintain the lifeline of patient care service in the police force hospitals. The service rendered by them is praiseworthy. Although many of them are still not combatised, they work shoulder to shoulder with regular police forces all the time and every where. In some forces, the combatisation of hospital staff has been effected much later than that of doctors. Some of them have not opted for khaki uniform and continue to be civilian staff for reasons best known to them. Of course, all new recruitments are for combatised service only. Apparently the most non-acceptable term of combatisation for the hospital staff is the reduction in the retirement age from 58 years to 55 years, at par with their police counter parts. Now, in the days of high cost of living no employee is prepared to lose a valuable period of three years from his service at the height of his career and emolument.

Any hospital runs its service by the help of large variety of workers. Like medical science itself, the workers of every branch and sub-branch needs some degree of expert hands to operate. In addition to the hospital staff there is another large group of behind-the-scene workers who also largely contribute to the smooth functioning of the medical services. They are the cooks, *safai karmacharis*, telephone operators, electricians, A.C. plant operator, plumber, generator operators, ambulance and staff car drivers and so on. The role of these staff is no way underrated. Although many of them belong to different departments like CPWD, motor transport division, Signabattalion, etc, they work in full co-ordination like a well-oiled machinery. They are the actual green room boys who manage the show beyond the eyes of the public.

While the doctors remain busy in clinical, administrative, public health or other job the work of the hospital and ancillary staff is co-ordinated by the Matron or the Sister In-charge, who in-turn reports to the Senior Medical Officer or Administrative Officer. He controls the functioning of each and every branch and ensures smooth running of patient care system with missionary zeal.

7

Role of Hospitals in Police Force Set-up

Hospitals, since centuries have institutionalised health care and thrive with the common motto--"Service to man is service to God", irrespective of the School of Medicine they follow. These institutions all over the world have undergone revolutionary changesin their layout, buildings, investigation and treatment facilities, sterilization, dis-aster management equipments, surgical and super speciality surgical manipulations. The thorough reforms and advancements specially in the branches like antibiotics, blood transfusion, accident management etc, are believed to be partly due to the two World Wars in the earlier half of the twentieth century.

But, hospitals of modern world are not only the magnificient architectural monuments or confined to the world of "ills and pills", but have developed as centres of multiferious social and welfare activities. The hospitals are now being used as health-clubs, physio-therapy and occupational therapy centres, dieting and fitness guiding centres, universal immunization agencies, vocational and rehabilitation guidance, etc. in addition to their normal curative duties. Field service of preventive and public health medicine have brought out the medical experts from their stuffy consultation chambers and have benefitted the mass, living beyond the vicinity of hospitals. The family planning activities have far reaching consequences to the community. The education on nutritional, hygiene and first-aid aspects have made the hospitals as the centre of disseminating the current medical knowledge among the general public. The blood donation camps, the relief operations during cyclone, flood and accidents have been well appreciated by all sections of press, public and the administrators. Such activities are ways of life in police force hospitals. The public service rendered by the field units of armed police force medical elements, in the far flung areas where no other medical aid are available have been well appreciated by the local administration. It would not be out of place to say that the author himself has visited large number of villages on the hills of North Tripura, trecking through the dense forests in all adversities of climate, leeches and militancy. These have been places in our country where the population remains far away from the light of civilization and have literally never seen a doctor. The author has the credit to visit such places in the early seventies in the Sakhan and Jampui hill ranges of Tripura.

Now, it is the fag end of twentieth century, when it is a waste to emphasise the role of any hospital in the community. Medical and health services have been the basic need and promise of the administration to the people. With the decade long planning and best efforts, the government has been able to provide the basic health care facilities to the masses. The national programme of "Health for All by 2000 AD" has to be achieved by all out efforts in the government and non-government levels. The departmental hospitals such as army hospitals, CPO hospitals, ESI and Railway hospitals and others, which are meant to look after the beneficiaries of their own department, promote the health environment of their own organisation as well as the country as a whole. Particularly, in the police force hospitals where the entire medical set-up is engaged in the maintenance of health, fitness and general physical and mental wellbeing of the trained manpower have a vital role to play in country's defence and internal security. Historical facts reveal that wars are lost or won based on the health standard of troops. The captive health set up is inevitable for the ever vigilant police forces fighting against heavy odds, reducing the morbidity and mortality rate in these forces.

Although it is not exhaustive, some of the basic functions of armed police force hospitals are discussed in the following paragraphs. The Medical Inspection Room, (called as M.I. Room) is the functional medical unit of a field unit. It is in-charge of a doctor and when not posted, looked after by a senior pharmacist. All the correspondence on medical and health matters are done through the in-charge of the medical unit. The role of hospitals or field unit are described under the following headings.

(a) Curative Role

The curative aspect covers providing treatment facilities to the members of force and their dependants. The force members are identified through their force number, dress, medical history sheet or record in sick report register, where as the dependants are issued with "Medical Benefit Cards" to claim facilities in the force hospitals. In absence of such card, they are introduced by any hospital staff or other force members. This restriction is enforced to restrict free flow of civilian patients to force hospitals leading to security lapse and community health hazards. Out Patient (OPD) treatment is available in every medical centre commonly, however small it may be, along with dispensing of drugs from the store. Patients can purchase any drug advised to them but not supplied from the hospital and the cost of the same is re-imbursed through essentiality certificate under Medical Attendance Rule. Laboratory investigations of routine nature are ordinarily carried in the hospitals when such facilities exist. In Battalion M.I. Rooms, the investigations are conducted by the doctor himself or arranged from the nearby civil hospital or private clinic. Wherever there is an established hospital, such facilities are bound to exist. Any test which may not be possible to conduct are done from outside hospitals as facilities like X-Ray, screening are available only in limited centres.

When the hospital maintains an indoor-ward, patients are admitted for isolation, observation, full rest and complete and continuous care. When the required specialists are posted, the operation theatre and labour room are also maintained. The indoor patients are provided with full nursing care, clean linen and hospital diet at government cost at an authorised scale. Free food is not supplied to officers drawing higher emoluments but partly supplied in tuberculosis and cancer cases. The patients who require treatment or investigations of higher nature, which may be beyond the scope of that hospital are referred to the better status hospitals of own force, other sister organisations or even any other hospital with formal approval from Chief Administrative Medical Officer or Medical Director as the case may be. In such cases, the cost of travel of patient, attendant and the hospital charges are borne by government. If the condition of the patient happens to be serious, the referring hospital may detail one doctor or para-medical staff to accompany upto the referal centre to provide emergency treatment enroute. Patient whose life is at risk are declared to be in "Seriously Ill List" (S.I.L.) and his next of kin informed by fastest means possible. Patients whose illness is thought to be potentially dangerous to the community are declared to be in "Dangerously Ill List" (D.I.L.).

In addition to the maintaining of a perfect patient care system, hospitals provide medical cover to visiting dignitaries, training camps, games and sports events which are integral part of every police force.

(b) Administrative Role

'Hospital administration' is itself a full length subject covering all aspects of smooth running of hospital and health services. But the topic is beyond the scope of this book. The administrative jobs to run a police hospital are looked after by the posted doctors themselves. In bigger hospitals like the

Base Hospitals, with authorised bed strength of 100 or above, one administrative officer is posted to upkeep the service, supply, maintenance, accounts, movement control, health transport, official correspondence, etc. While other doctors are busy in caring for the suffering.

The most common administrative job performed by these hospitals is the conducting of Medical Board to judge the suitability of members of force after injury or prolonged illness for active police duties. It involves the terminal disposal of a member of force, who suffered from prolonged illness attributable to his nature of duties, operational or accidental injuries and has received the full course of treatment. Inspite of the complete possible treatment, the individual is not likely to prove to be an efficient member of the police force. The case is first documented and board is composed. The board should include a specialist of the concerned disease for which the member of force is being examined. In some hospitals, there is a standing Medical Board, consisting of a physician, an orthopedic surgeon and an ophthalmologist, presided over by the Senior-most among them. The commanding officer acts on the basis of recommendation of the medical board, with guidelines from service rules.

Vocational guidance and rehabilitative measures are also offered to persons with partial incapacity, who cannot perform the hard duty of a policeman but can be useful in any other field of less laborious nature. If the authorities agree, the service of such person can be utilised as a welfare measure, to help him earn his livelihood in addition to the nominal pension.

The force hospitals deal with a variety of cases, some of them are really problematic. Among the police patients, a sizable number are malingerers. The malingerer's are healthy or not so ill persons, pretending illness to get excuse from work. Police patients are privileged to get excuse from P.T. Parade, night duty, boot or belt excuse or sometimes complete rest on the recommendation of doctor, without affecting their emolument or leave. But such malingering is a misconduct. When such cases are detected, the policeman is liable to be punished.

More of malingering cases come up with the wake of strong operational duties, transfers to faraway places away from the family station and duties of hazardous and unpleasant nature. Most of the illnesses reported by this group of patients are of vague nature but with such description that the medical staffs are misled. Inspite of the doubt, on the genuinity of the illness, the medical team has to conduct all investigation and institute all possible treatment in fear of neglecting a genuine illness, not apparently diagnosed. All investigations, results in such cases are normal or inconclusive and all treatments seem failed. The patient tries to avoid treatment but exaggerates his symptoms. Pain in abdomen, chest, back, or legs, are the commonly observed complaints. Out right rejection of their complaints is not possible by doctors as they find difficulty to establish evidence in support of their opinion and the humanitarian consideration. These patients describe their illness with serious note on first reporting, while being observed and try to avoid taking drugs. They behave normally when not being watched. They are afraid of treatment with injections and oppose to any surgical procedure. It is interesting to note that some police families feign illness to draw sympathy from the commanders of their menfolk and get excuse from hard duty, delay or cancel transfers. Exacerbation of old ailment is common pattern of police family malingering on the wake of hardship in service line. Such cases cause undue harassment to the medical staff, consume hospital resources and waste technical time.

Other bafling cases causing administrative bottle-neck to the police medical officers are the psychopathic or mentally ill case, alcoholics and the drug addicts. These cases form the index of the deteriorating disciplinary standard in forces. Such cases need utmost care and strict vigilance. The disposal needs co-ordination of medical and administrative care-takers.

(c) Preventive Role

The police force hospitals follow the international norm by maintaining well--child clinics in the family stations for universal immunisation of children upto six years of age. The expectant mothers are also immunised against preventable diseases in the ante-natal check ups. Every member of force is immunised against cholera and TAB, every year. During basic training of recruits and drivers, they are prone to injury by metallic parts of vehicles and weapons. Hence, they are protected with Tetanus toxoid in full prophylaxis doses, in addition to its use after injury and surgical procedures. With total global eradication of smail pox, the administration of its vaccine is discontinued. The camp population of a police force cantonment is fully protected by regular immunization.

The food handlers like cook, water carriers, mess boys, milk supplier, water truck man, soda fountain operators and Canteen servers are periodically inspected and deworming done by oral administration of anthelminth drugs. This helps in eradication of carriers and prevention of epidemics. The hospital staff specially those who work in operation theatre, casualty section, labour room and clinical laboratory handle blood, serum, saliva and human excreta. They are at constant risk to contact diseases like Hepatitis-B and need to be protected against it by suitable vaccine. Although the risk is equally deadly for AIDS, no anti-HIV vaccine so far has been developed. Dog-bite cases are fully immunised by anti-rabic vaccine. Killing of street dogs which hang around the kitchen area are taken up periodically with help of municipal anti-dog squad.

(d) Public Health Role

Indian police forces have adopted the sanitary inspection system in army pattern. The unit medical officer periodically inspects the camp, cook houses, barracks, disposal of garbage system, water supply plant, etc. and reports with suggestions for improvement to the commanding officer. In larger stations where the senior-most medical officer acts as the Station Health Officer, undertakes periodic inspection of vulnerable points of health hazards. Areas like family lines, butchery, Canteen, ration stores are given special attention. He issues notifications and warnings to all unit heads regarding spread of epidemics in addition to informing the local municipal health officer, district medical officer and own directorate.

Anti-fly measures, anti-mosquito measures, case finding of Malaria carriers, periodic chemical analysis of drinking water and disinfection of water sources are routinely done in police forces. Upkeeping of camp sanitation in the best possible state is the aim and endeavour of doctors and station commander. On the detection of any communicable disease case, the necessary precautions are taken alerting all the camp dwellers. Police camps in past have been in the clutch of epidemics like gastro-entrities, meningitis, hepatitis and chicken pox besides the rampant cases of malaria. Because of barrack life and common kitchen, the spread of epidemic is rapid. Hence, prompt action only helps in the prevention of loss of lives and loss of man-days. In the malaria endemic zones, cases of cerebral malaria lead to undue toll of life. When a policeman contacts any disease during the course of duty, he is entitled to get all the official sickness benefits during and after treatment and convalescence period. Loss of trained man-power presses heavily on the national economy.

(e) Health Education

Health education to the troops is dealt in detail in other chapters of this book. Health education is a part of the curriculum in every training programme in military and para-military forces even in NCC, Homeguards, Village Volunteer Force, Scouts and Guides, etc. Non-government associations like Rastriya Swayam Sevak Sangh (RSS) also impart training of first-aid, sanitations, personal hygiene, sex education, effects of smokings, alcoholism, benefits of small family and ideal ways of child-care, etc. Officers' academies have elaborate arrangements for lecture by expert guests in different fields.

Health guidance or education is a continuous process. Doctors keep on advising their beneficiaries on health "dos" and "don'ts" in their day to day hospital work. The presence of their own medical cadre officers is helpful in continuous advice at formal and informal occasions. Such practice cannot be ensured when doctors are engaged in part time, leave reserve, visiting or locum basis or when taken on deputation from State Governments. The units can plan training programmes for men specially, first aid training to drivers, auto-fitters, and armourers.

Teaching aids like charts, slides, over-head projectors, movies, video and audio cassettes on health education topics are used to make the instructions more appealing, illustrative and lively. Barracks, hospitals, recreation rooms, canteens and other public places bear display of posters for repeated hammering of educative points in the minds of policemen.

The doctors and para-medical staff who serve as instructors need to refresh their knowledge and improve their instructional capability. Medicine is an ever expanding science and its horizon widens continuously, in matters of diagnosis, treatment, teaching, research and bio-medical equipments. They attend and organise medical conferences, seminars and symposiums, group discussions among themselves and in the nearby hospitals. Occasional film-shows and video display on medical topics are also arranged. Some of the pharmaceutical manufacturers circulate showing of video films of their products to doctors and hospital staffs. Such programmes can be arranged periodically. Guest lectures by eminent speakers are also educative.

(f) Family Welfare

The national policy of small family norm is also required to be implemented in the police force personnel to combat the population explosion. The subject is already over emphasised by all the media in the country. It is highly relevant to think for implementation of this and other national policies in the forces for two reasons Firstly, they are the "Controlled Groups" of population, over whom the government has good control and take benefit of their disciplined behaviour in the greater interest of the nation. Secondly, the police force hospitals have abundant free medical facilities within their reach and can motivate and operate on the eligible couples. The health visitors and other field staff like social workers can spot the eligible couples and educate them to accept permanent methods of family planning. Even cases among the women police force and the woman wing of the Home Guards, can be spotted and brought to hospital for advice, etc. Candidates do not report to hospitals for family welfare methods due to ignorance, lack of motivation, misconception of after effects of operation, single male child, consecutive girl child deliveries etc. This can be eradicated by imparting proper education to them and by giving convincing replies to their querries and reassuring them.

In addition to case motivation, mass education programmes like lectures in assembly of families, troops, exhibition, demonstration and film-shows on the subject be arranged. District Family Planning Unit or State Directorate of Family Welfare may be able to lend extensive support on such moves. Family planning fortnight is observed twice a year. During this period, family planning operation drive with ample incentives to acceptors should be organised so that more and more eligible and willing couples can be brought into the society of small family.

As already discussed, the health and moral of Police Force directly affects the work out-put and effective policing. Conversely, the size of policeman's family directly affects his health, changing his life style and retarding his active duty. A policeman with limited salary has to meet all expenditure for his family, fulfil the social obligations and also save for the future. In this situation the burden of large family leads to fall in standard of living, lack of adequate and nutritive food, chronic sickness and lassitude, mental tension, economic bankruptcy and unhappiness. All these ill effects of large family has direct effect on his performance as an efficient and alert member of the police force. He cannot be expected to maintain a sound physique and tension free mind which is of utmost importance in active police duty.

(g) Philanthropic Role

Swami Vivekananda had once called upon the youth of the country to come forward for nation's building in the following words. "My brave lads, have courage of a lion and spirit of a philanthropist". What the Indian Police Forces are doing today or their medical set-up is observing as part of their routine duty is nothing but "Nation Building" in plain words. Without their presence, the unity and integrity both in geographical, emotional, religious and other sense is impossible. Hence, a high degree of devotion, sacrifice and Spirit of the philanthropist is absolutely necessary to perform the great task of nation building and thereby be a successful member of police force justifying the saying of Swamiji. This philosophy has been rightly chosen to decide the motto of some major police organisations, such as "Service and Loyalty" (CRPF) and "Service unto Death", (BSF) and the members now to translate the concept to action.

As discussed earlier, the century old image of police forces have been inherited from their feudal past. It has been the arm of the ruling government against criminals and law-breakers. But police forces have put human touch in such action also. In moments of flood, draught, cyclone, train accidents, earth-quacks, devastating fire the men in arms have come forward to help the marooned in rebuilding their houses, providing food, temporary shelter, distribution of clothings, etc. The medical team deputed to the area deliver more useful service of treating the population, and saving them from epidemics in a number of ways. The dedication and devotion of police force medical teams are commendable.

In the "peace time" also, the hospitals are engaged in various benevolent activities such as organising eye check-up camps, blood-donation camps, first-aid to civilians, providing medical cover in mela, fairs, festivals, etc. Some units adopt villages and look into the health, education, sanitation, family planning, nutritional supplement of the villagers, school children and expectant mothers. Repair of old roads, repair of school building and disinfection of ponds and wells are taken up as voluntary service. The police force hospitals render services much beyond the hospital premises and perimeters of their well-guarded campuses.

(h) Surveillance and Quarantine Service

The police force hospitals as a matter of their routine duties perform few surveillance and quarantine services which are of significance. The annual medical check-up of all the members of police forces, the periodic eye, hearing and mental alertness check up of automobile drivers, the quarterly deworming and inspection of cooks and other food handlers, nutritional and health survey of Montessory school and other school children of the campus are some of the surveillance services. This activity helps in early detection of any active pathological and psychological negative effect and check further deterioration by timely action.

Persons who come back after long outing like camping, training course, leave, escorting prisoners and patients and after known exposure like industrial pollution etc. are tested for harbouring any potentiality communicable disease serves as the quarantine duties of police hospitals. The quarantine services are of more practical and scientific nature in approach. The suspected persons are isolated and waited till a reasonable incubation period is passed. After suffering from infectious diseases, the person is not allowed to stay in the unit lines during convalescence and infectivity period. He is granted leave on medical ground with full benefits of pay, ration allowance, etc. and issued with free railway pass to visit his home town. Persons reporting from the endemic malaria zone are tested for their carrier State.

The readers may feel that the role of police force hospitals of the country described in this chapter are none so unique as any hospital, more or less run under similar motto and philosophy. But it is not unusual to say the obvious truth that the degree of moral values and humanitarian consideration of professionals have eroded all over the world. The ethics and Hippocratic oaths which has preserved the service mentality of the health professionals and institutions through centuries have undergone thorough degeneration and degradation. But the police force hospitals are the only few such institutions which are proudly maintaining the dignity of profession, devoted in performing all its role, honest to the core, in the benefit of the suffering mass. It would not be as exaggeration to say that they are the only such group of hospitals, conscious in maintaining higher human values in the country. Quoting few words from Charaka would be a fitting tribute to the great sage of Medicine-

"No other gift is greater than the gift of life. The patient may doubt his relatives, his sons, and even his parents, but he has full faith in his physician. He gives himself up in the doctor's hands, and has no misgivings about him. Therefore, it is the physician's duty to look after him as his own".

8

Medical Arrangements in Police Formations

The incorporation of the medical element in the composition of police forces traditionally, speaks of health consciousness of the troop commanders and attaching enough importance to healthy living and fitness of troops. Although the armed police forces have basically different roles to play, at time they have to remain under operational control of army, working shoulder to shoulder with them. On the International frontiers the BSF and ITBP have to be in close communication with the army units of the area even without being operationally under their command. The CRPF operates in close correlation with army in counter insurgency operations. The Assam Rifles has the organic link with army for operational purpose and has reasons to follow the army medical pattern as the basic frame-work in their medical care system. The Armed Constabulary, Military Police, Special Armed Police Forces, India Reserve Battalions of different States and the Civil Police formations who draw their medical facilities from the local police hospitals follow more of a civil hospital pattern rather than the military or para-military pattern in the health services.

The medical facilities provided and the arrangements designed in the different formations of police forces is with the pre-conceptions that they deal with basically a healthy group of population and the medical set-up is meant to back up the emergency requirements in operational situations, accidents, natural calamities and regimental purposes. Moreover, the presence of medical branch providing basic health care facilities, keep the moral of the force high. A good medical service is one of the major welfare measure the unit can provide to its men and their families. A hospital or medical aid centre, small or big, in the field area is the source of consolation, encouragement and inspiration for the hard working policemen when they are down with disease or injury. Men who sacrificed their youth, comfort and best years of life in the service in police forces with courage and bravery but unfortunately get incapacitated in action, draw their benefits through hospitals.

The medical facilities provided in police forces can be discussed broadly under two headings such as Field Formation Service and the Peace Unit Hospital Services.

(a) The Field Medical Service

The smallest medical element attached with a duty battalion is called the Medical Inspection Room (M.I. Room) or unit hospital or field hospital. In some forces it works like a first-aid post or field ambulance service. A "Battalion" is the smallest functional unit in a police force under unitary command comprising of five to six service companies, and a Headquarter Command module regulating the administrative and operational affairs of all the companies. In a battalion, one or two doctors are posted with some para-medical staff. In CPOs, each battalion M.I. Room is supposed to maintain a 10 bedded hospital in the battalion headquarters. In ITBP and Assam Rifles, where the deployment is wide-spread, each service company is provided with doctors and para-medical staff. In forces other than CRPF, the small hospitals in battalion level is thriving with functional capability to meet the requirement because of permanent and semi-permanent location of battalion headquarters. But in CRPF, it is possible only when the unit has a permanent or semi-permanent battalion headquarter with adequate facilities like accommodation. Otherwise, a M.I. Room runs, providing only first-aid and OPD services. Cases requiring hospitalization, long treatment, higher investigation, surgery, etc. are referred to nearby police hospital, civil hospitals, or medical college hospital. The hospital of choice should always be the hospital of one's own organization. But in emergency cases, the nearest hospital is preferred to save the life and save the unit from suffering of loss of man-days.

When the service companies are deployed at far flung places, where medical facilities are not available to men easily, a pharmacist with common medicines and first-aid field dressing materials is engaged to provide medical cover. Any person requiring better medical attention is sent to the battalion headquater or the visit of a Medical Officer is requisitioned.

The most common hardship of keeping the medical service system in tact in a duty battalion is the frequent movement of the unit. When the law and order situation improves and the services of the Central para-military forces are not required, the forces move out of the place and rush to another hot spot. Such situations are almost a part of day to day life in CRPF and BSF. Even when the unit moves in a special train from one part of the country to another, the medical branch continues to render first-aid and OPD service during the movement.

The medical officer in-charge serves as the advisor to the commanding officer in the matters of public health hygiene and sanitation and forms a part of the group in the unit caring for the welfare of men and their dependants. All other duties are already discussed in other chapters. The medical service at the battalion level is the real heart and soul of police medical service, for it serves the active policemen in the fields, exposed to all adversities of climates, casualties and accidents. The majority of the policemen comprise in this category. Hence, as a healthy practice, the service should be continuous and provisioning should be adequate.

(b) The Field Unit Hospital Services

The idea of creating hospital, exclusively for police personnel is one of the successful need based experiment in the pre-independent India. By this the occasional medical service taken for prisoners in jail, in police interrogations, torture-cells or capital punishment has been made permanent and continuous. The service was further extended to Reserve Police Force lines and has gradually taken the shape of full time hospitals. The Armed Wings of State Police were looked after by doctors deputed by the civil surgeon on request of the District Superintendent of Police or Deputy Inspector General.

The Central police forces have their independent medical set-up, who run their own chain of hospitals in different parts of the country. Some of the large sized hospitals are designated as "Base Hospital" which serve as the referal hospitals and provide supplementary medical care not possible in field M.I. Rooms or smaller hospitals. Permanent centres with built up campus like group centres, training centres, training colleges, academies, ordinance depots, motor transport service centres, signal and technical centres, record offices, data processing and accounting units, etc. have permanent hospitals in all the forces. The hospital is normally headed by a senior medical officer with administrative experience for over all control of all the sections of health care deliveries. The doctors form a mixed group of specialists and non-specialists complementing and supplementing each others' work. A well established hospital has to provide the basic amenities of patient care, dispensary service, Indoor ward, labour room, operation theatre, dressing and plaster service, Laboratory, X-Ray, ECG facilities, etc. Some hospitals are also equipped with physio-therapy and acupuncture units. The available facilities cater to the needs of force members and their families to a reasonable extent, except in some rare occasions when the patient is referred out for any special investigation or treatment.

The Senior Medical Officer in-charge of the hospital has to maintain good liaison with the nearby civil and police hospitals and District Medical Officer for various clinical and administrative purposes. The Army Hospitals, of course, extend facilities to police patients only when the unit is under their operational control. When more number of units and institutions are situated at the same station, a "Central Hospital" or "Station Hospital" is formed by amalgamating the medical elements of all the units and entrusted in the health care activities. A Station Co-ordination Committee comprising heads of all units, doctors, local health officers and municipal medical authority periodically review the functioning and suggest improvement. The medical officer in-charge of station hospital becomes the Member-Secretary. Representation of all sections of beneficiaries including women members is ensured.

The story of these hospitals, though not very old, has been always a happy one. They have proved remarkable success and have an impact in the society.

Treatment in Base Hospitals

The base hospitals are independent units headed by a Chief Medical Officer (CMO) situated in a large centre of police activities. State police forces do not maintain any base hospital but large size police hospitals are established in places like Calcutta and Madras. It is only the Central Para-military forces who partially follow the army like pattern of hospitals, have established base hospitals in busy centres. The size of the base hospitals, is around 100 bed strong and serve as the referal centre of all other small hospitals and the duty battalion M.I. Rooms. The staffing is designed to cater to all major specialisation equipped with modern equipments of diagnosis and treatment. Indoor facilities with isolation ward, mental disease ward, T.B. Ward, officers ward and mortury are the extra addition in base hospitals after the common para-phrenalia. Sophisticated investigations like ultra-sonography, Trade-mill test, Echo-cardiography and Endoscopy are also performed at some centres. Almost all routine surgical, gynaecological, orthopedic and Eye ENT Surgeries are conducted at all the base hospitals. CPO hospitals are not yet equipped and experienced to undertake neurosurgical and cardiothoracic surgery cases in own hospitals. Treatment in such cases is arranged in the advanced centres, the cost of which is duly re-imbursed.

The day to day administration, service, supply, sanitation, movement of patients, health transport system, etc. are looked after by one of the senior doctors who is designated as the Administrative Officer of the hospital. He usually possesses a special degree on Hospital Administration and enough experience to keep the hospital in exemplary state in all respect.

Although not designated as Base Hospital, quite a good number of big hospitals are also run by the E.S.I. (Employees State Insurance) Corporation where the men of CISF get treatment along with the industrial workers. Besides, the railway has fairly good hospitals where members of Government Railway Police and Railway Protection Force (RPF) are treated. The public sector undertakings run their own hospitals in the factory premises, labour colonies and mining sites. They extend basic medical services to the men of CISF on duty in their locality.

The Base Hospitals of CPOs and the Upgraded hospitals of other organizations function as regional centres for diagnosis, treatment and rehabilitation of sick police personnels. They co-ordinate movement from the field units to the base hospitals and non-police medical centres. Contact with local and advance medical centres are affected through these hospitals for higher treatment in deserving cases. The CMO or SMO takes the responsibility of arranging his treatment in any other hospital in the country. There have been instances, when a particular drug was unavailable in the country, the same has been imported through the concerned foreign embassy and the drug had made available to the patient at government cost.

Air evacuation of patients from the operational areas to the suitable hospitals by contacting the Army and Civil Aviation authorities has been proved life-saving in most cases. The BSF also maintains its own Air-wing which lifts patients from remote border operating posts (BOPs) for all the forces under CPO, particularly, evacuation of personnels severely injured in gun battle, accident, bomb-blast in J & K, Nagaland, Mizoram, Tripura and Arunachal Pradesh when other modes of transport were not available or delayed, which may have risked the patients life.

Base hospitals are centres for active academic and research activities. Maintenance of a good library and video facilities is part of continuing education programme for the senior doctors and preparatory for higher studies for young ambitious doctors. A general library also caters for issuing books to interested patients to read during their hospital stay. The benefits of library are enjoyed also by nursing staff, para-medical staff, trainees undergoing combatisation, First-aid Course and families staying in hospital premises.

Treatment in Army and Other Hospitals

As stated earlier, the army hospital treat patients from police forces only in operational areas, injured in action and accidents. They take up "Cold Surgery" and other cases only in emergency and relieve them for convalescence and further follow-up in own force hospitals. In the Kashmir valley, the army hospitals have been doing commendable job by extending full co-operation to all police forces. Conversely, the police hospitals of State or Central Police formations, gladly allow the army and allied forces patients for treatment under information to the concerned army unit, without any charge for cost of treatment.

The patients of police forces requiring treatment of advanced nature such as Anti-cancer treatment, Cardio-thoracic surgery, Neuro-surgical operations, Laser treatment, Keratoplasty, Prosthesis and artificial limb etc. are referred to hospitals where such treatment may be available. In such cases, the cost of treatment is very high and beyond the scope of a policeman. The cost is met by liberal grant from the Central welfare and benevolent fund. The Medical Officer In-charge of the referring hospital acts as the authorised medical attendant. In case of death of a patient, the dependants are well looked after by granting liberalised pension to the next of kin, ex-gratia payment and offering employment to any of the eligible dependant, qualifying for any post in the force. Benefits of risk fund and group insurance are made available on priority basis.

Procurement of Hospital Stores

Every hospital needs constant supply of huge quantity of stores of divergent nature. The principal items of store are medicines, equipments, linen, furnitures, diet articles, etc. In bigger hospitals, a permanent service and supply department is engaged in the regular replenishment of exoendable items, planning, budgeting, repair of unserviceable tems and their disposals. In addition, they also take care of water-supply, electricity, air-conditioning system, disposal of hospital refuges, safeguarding of hospital properties, repair and replacement of old furnitures, maintenance of telephone and inter-com service, etc. But in smaller hospitals as in CPO, a pharmacist or a procurement clerk is engaged in the job.

Medical Stores

The medical store includes not only a long list of drugs and pharmaceuticals, but also allied items like syringe, needle, dressing and bandage items, I.V. Sets, laboratory and X-Ray chemicals, oxygen cylinders, surgical instruments, sterilizing equipments, gloves, etc. The bulk supply of drugs and hospital items are procured by all government hospitals from the government Medical Stores Depots (MSD) situated at Karnal, Delhi, Calcutta, Guwahati, Madras and Bombay. The MSD in close proximity is preferred to avoid delay in transport and heavy cost of freight charges. The depots also supply surgical instruments and O.T. equipments, anaesthetic items, sterilization equipments and ECG machines on special demands. In case any of the stores is not supplied, the same are procured from the market after observing complete purchase formalities and financial sanction from competent authority. Unnecessary over stocking of store is avoided and in case of over stocking of any of the items, it is transferred to needy units before expiry date, to ensure in-time utilization to avoid loss of government store and harassment to needy patients.

General Stores

There are a large number of general (non-medical) items required in the day to day functioning of hospitals. The most significants out of them are furnitures, mattresses, linens, patients dress, cleaning detergents, hygiene and sanitation items, heating and cooling electrical gadgets, stationery items, books and periodicals, and several others. In police force hospitals most of the general store items are supplied from the stores of the battalion, Group Centres or the parent police organisation of the station. The budgeting on this heads being liberal, such items can be made available to hospital in plenty with meticulous planning.

Diet to Police Patients

The police patients upto a particular pay range are authorised free diet while admitted in hospital. The diet slip is prepared and sent to diet section one day in advance. The types of diet are categorised and advised by the treating physician. Grossly, the category of diets are Ordinary Diet (Veg or Non-veg), T.B. Diet (Veg or Non-veg) Fluid Diet, Convalescent Diet, Diabetic Diet, etc. The physician may further specify his desire of diet as per illness of the patient such as salt free diet, fat free diet and so on. The scale of ration articles in each type of diet is laid down in the manual. The food prepared in the kitchen is distributed among the patients in two principal meals. Lunch and Dinner, Breakfast and Tea, daily. The ration articles are procured from unit co-operative shop or from approved suppliers. Fresh ration like vagetable, meat, fish, milk are purchased daily and dry category articles, are purchased for a week. The cost of the ration is met from the advance available with the medical officer in-charge and the bills are periodically sent to pay and accounts office for re-imbursement after financial sanction from head of the office.

Usually one under office is in-charge of the section for procurement of ration, supervise distribution of diet, and keeping accounts of expenditure. He is assisted by one or two constables and the authorised number of cooks. The doctors and nursing staff periodically check the food for its quality, teste, use of cooking medium, cleanliness and timely service. A high standard of food in all respect can be maintained as there is no restriction on the amount of expenditure. Mess staff are advised to use proper cleaning agents and warm water for washing of utensils to avoid cross infection.

Line Committee and Classification Board

In the purchase and disposal of stores of any nature, a laid down procedure is followed in all police forces. The same order is applicable to the hospital also. When any store is purchased, a board of officers is detailed to check the quality, quantity, expiry date and serviceability of the store. The board expresses its view on a particular proforma. It is called the "Line-Committee Report". The committee may reject any article assigning the reasons. They are to note the extent of shortage, damage or pilferage of store.

The used up and unserviceable items of hospital are displayed before a duly constituted "Classification Board" and the board is to declare any items produced before it to be either, unserviceable or resume. Unserviceable items are sent to general store for auction. These procedures are time tested and has been found useful to avoid any malpractice in the store affairs.

Health Transport Service

Health transport system in police forces are managed from the large number of ambulance vans and other vehicles supplied to hospitals. The vehicles are parked around the hospital and the doctor on emergency duty acts as the Motor Transport Officer (MTO) of the vehicle, who approves plying of vehicles on requisition by any hospital staff or patients attendant. The Senior Medical Officer in-charge of the hospital counter signs the care diary formally. The posting of drivers, the supply of Fuel and lubricating Oil, repair and servicing of vehicles, etc. are done by the police office of the station. Any vehicle going "Off road" for technical reason is replaced with suitable alternative and repair work is taken upon priority basis.

The use of police ambulance can be summarised as follows:

1. To carry the doctor on emergency duty in non-hospital hours from his residence to hospital to attend emergency calls, and return to his residence after treatment, operation, delivery, etc.

2. Carrying patients to outside hospitals referred by the medical officers of police hospital for specialist consultation, special investigation, advance treatment, etc.

3. Carrying patients transferred from army or civil hospitals after treatment for convalescence in police hospital.

4. In law and order duties, the ambulance is kept as a stand-by to carry any injured policemen to hospital for first-aid and treatment.

5. Transfer of criminals, prisoners, undertrials from jail, *hazat* (Police Custody) to police hospital or any other hospital on their illness for treatment.

6. Patients required to be transported to a hospital beyond the city limit or outside district when the condition of patients is such that they cannot travel by public transport. Such patients are shifted by police ambulance. When the condition demands, even a doctor or para-medical staff along with attendant may accompany to provide medical cover enroute.

7. The benevolent and philanthropic duties performed by police ambulance in the carriage of civilians wounded in the incident to the nearest hospital.

8. In sports events, the accompanying or on duty police ambulance provides transport to the injured, drop-outs from game and persons suddenly falling ill such as fainting, stroke, dehydration, palpitation or breathlessness, drowning, survivor of burn, etc. while performing sports or rescue activities.

As a general rule, any vehicle available can be used as ambulance in emergency but use of designed ambulance for other purposes is restricted. Particularly carriage of dead body should be avoided in an ambulance as subsequent cleaning and disinfection becomes cumbersome due to the emergency fittings.

As a general overview, the medical arrangements in police hospitals, particualrly, the CPO hospitals are of complete satisfactory standard. The story of these hospitals, though not very old, always has been a happy one. They have proved to be a remarkable success and have had a tremendous impact on the societv

9

Evaluation of Traditions and Procedures

In post-Independent era, Indian Police Forces have undergone a sea change. Older forces like the Central Reserve Police Force (CRPF) and the Assam Rifles have rapidly grown in size and structure, as new forces like Border Security Forces (BSF), Central Industrial Security Force (CISF), Indo-Tibetan Border Police (ITBP), National Security Guard (NSG), etc. have been created for specialised jobs. In every state, the armed police wings have also expanded their strength and auxillary forces like the Home Guards, Village Volunteer force etc. have been raised for reinforcement of police strengths on disturbed law and order situation. The increasing incidence of communal riots and insurgency in various parts of the country, which the local armed police forces failed to control required Central assistance. Hence, the Central Forces have to supplement State Police Forces besides continuing their supportive role to regular army in maintaining vigilance over the international frontier. The malignant growth of these forces has forced a thorough reorganisation of their set-up from administrative and operational point of view.

Every organisation has its own systems and procedures in every branch and areas. The police forces also follow a few procedures in medical matters. If the history of each systems is traced back, some of them are indigenous and others are copied from the Indian Army, i.e., the Army Medical Corp (AMC). The systems have gone through a thorough metamorphosis on transition with passage of time, to suit to the requirement of police forces whose role is different from that of an army. The reasons for following a modified army pattern are firstly, due to the influx of large number of army officers, subordinate officers, and *sipahis* in the process of rehabilitation and to nucleate the rapidly growing forces and secondly, army is the only model available to follow where these systems have worked flawlessly for centuries. Even in the army, the systems and procedures have undergone metamorphosis through the ages and such changes are inevitable in police forces. Every para-military force has put its own colour and flavour to the system before serving it on the table of practice, like a cap adopts the shape of the head that wears it.

In the police force hospitals, the doctors and para-medical staff hold degrees and diplomas from Civil institutions. Hence, the basic principle and concept of patient care remains the same as any other hospital. But the procedures are to help the administration to maintain discipline, prevent self-doctoring and keeping the overall health standard in high profile. The executive branches of the police forces contain non-medical police personnel. The procedures are so devised that they are in full agreement to both sides. Some of the common procedures are like the sick report or sick parade, special sick report, annual medical inspection, periodic inspection of followers, test of special senses of drivers, health check-up of incoming and outgoing troops, pre-course fitness, health check-up of school children, hygiene and sanitation round of camp area, health reporting of officers etc. Although every system has its own pitfall and limitations, they have percolated through the generations of police forces. The working of some of these systems and procedures are analysed here.

1. Sick Report (Sick Parade) Systems

This is a very old system in all military and para-military forces. Any member of force falling sick and unable to perform duty assigned to him is to bring the fact to the notice of his immediate superior. The man is relieved from his duty by proper reliever and produced before the doctor in-charge of the battalion by his platoon or section commander. His nominal role particulars (Name, rank, force number, company, battalion, etc.) are entered to the sick report register. The doctor on duty examines him in the unit medical inspection room (M.I. Room). The doctor records his provisional diagnosis or chief symptom, gravity of sickness on the register. The method of categorisation of gravity of sickness is already laid down in rules. According to the category, the doctor recommends his rest, light duty or full duty for the day. The remark is valid for next 24 hours or next sick parade time, after which the condition is reviewed and fresh remark is endorsed. Some deserving cases are hospitalised or temporarily detained in the hospital. Cases not manageable in unit level are referred to the nearly hospital for better investigation and treatment.

Infact, the sick parade is taken up in the early hours of the day, with the beginning of the day's curriculum. Any member falling sick after this time are produced in "special sick report" and similar procedure is followed. But usually, those who skip the morning sick-report time are treated without any official record in OPD. Patients who suddently fall ill in odd hours of the day are brought in emergency and treated on priority basis without waiting for sick register, a formality which may follow later.

There are two basic concepts behind the sick report system. Firstly, the members of force can enjoy rest or duty of light nature on doctors recommendation without affecting his leave or emoluments. This is an advantage given by government to men of armed forces who work day and night far away from their native place separated from family and children. Secondly, the sickness of any trained soldier should be in full knowledge of his Commander who is responsible for his day to day life and duty, so that he arranges his reliever as well as his treatment. This is also to prevent loss of man-days by misuse of doctor's advice by the malingerers as to avoid hazardous duties, strenuous exercise and training programmes, sudden movements, long transfers, etc. The Commander has to plan his operational action as per the fit manpower available under his command. Hence, the philosophy behind this vital police-Medical procedure was absolutely practical, operation oriented and part of manpower planning and health care.

But as a general observation, the practice of the sick report system in police hospitals in States and Central para-military forces has been found to be full of defects. The hospitals treat large crowd of these troops but only 2-5% of them are in official sick report. This clearly means, men seek treatment in hospital for their ailments but avoid and bypass the sick report procedures. This has created a wrong notion in the minds of higher police authorities that the police hospitals have very scanty work, inspite of the really heavy work-load. Because the senior officers go by the official statistics on sick report, such impression is bound to be formed. Infact, the authorities and local Commander have indirectly allowed the 'off-record' treatment in view of shortage of man-power and only when some excuse is desired, proper procedure followed. A conservative study as to why men avoid to attend hospital through the official sick report and prefer to be treated without entering to official formalities has been made. Some of salient observations are listed below :

(a) Ignorance

The existence of such a procedure is not seriously taught to the troops in their basic training and hence the difference in the police hospital and civil hospital is not properly fed to their minds. As the current trend prevails, the facility through sick report systems is made available only to those requiring excuses. Hence, the systems and services of medical branch in a police force is used to the convenience and not as a regimental procedure. This anomaly can be remedied by proper knowledge of rules and health education.

(b) Hiding of Ailments

The illness of the troops in sick report is recorded in the official records like sick report register, medical history sheet and hospital records. Diseases like venereal diseases, skin disease and many other conditions may lead to departmental enquiries, punishments and bad service record. Hence, the troops try to avoid reporting full facts to the departmental doctors of force hospital. They prefer to get treated from private doctors or outside hospitals where departmental restrictions are ineffective.

(c) Economic Factor

The troops in the field areas get nominal detachment allowance daily as an incentive to work in forward and operational areas, physically and constructively. Such allowances are deducted when the man is admitted to hospital or advised rest. Men are afraid of such financial loss and hence, avoid sick report.

Thus, it cannot be pronounced finally that the system has outlived its utility but serves more of individual purpose rather than departmental or regimental purpose. The staff who should uphold the convention do not implement the system seriously. The doctors and medical branch are in the receiving end. They are wrongly blamed for inadequate work.

2. Annual Medical Examination

The entire medical care service of the force is devoted in keeping the standard of health and moral in his profile. In other words, the troops have to be kept 'fighting fit' all the time. As a matter of routine, all members of the force, even if apparently well, are subjected to undergo medical inspection. This procedure is followed in the army in the form of periodic medical inspection, sometimes every month. It may be possible for the army because their troops are probably deployed in close conteguity and the Unit Medical Officer has open excess to the entire battalion population. But in para-military forces, the troops are mostly deployed in far flung places, sometimes another end of the country or places not connected by vehicular traffic. Hence, only one inspection is possible every year by the long medical officer, with full documentation and reports to commanding officers. The system is still actively in practice in all police, para-military and auxillary forces though the degree of seriousness and official importance varies.

The aims of conducting the Annual Medical Examination for each force member are summarised below :

(a) The trained police forces help the government to run the administration smoothly. Hence, the loss of trained man-power by morbidity and mortality costs heavily on the public exchequer. The safe guarding of the health of the force is in the national interest.

(b) To diagnose and treat promptly any conspicuous ailment in the policemen-In case of suspicion, the man is referred to the concerned specialist and conduct required pathological, radiological and other investigation.

(c) To note the deterioration of health standard due to advancing of age. Although, these charges are inevitable, some persons undergo rapid ageing whereas other exhibit slow effect on their health. Proper record has to be maintained in respect of cardio-vascular respiratory function, effect of exercise, visual standard, state of limbs, etc. The serious deterioration of health standard may make him unsuitable for police duty with long march, sentry duty, night duty and operational duty, etc.

(d) Some diseases developing in latter part of life like varicosity of veins, herniation, cataract, etc. are treatable conditions. Presence of such diseases hampers the active duty hence, early treatment helps him to maintain normal life. The conditions hard to treat are tick, tumour, backache and arthritic diseases. Development of such condition interferes in duty.

(e) Assessment of mental functions. With the advance of age, liability, tension from family and pressure of duty, some persons develop serious deterioration of mental faculties and show signs of forgetfulness, error of judgement and incoherent talk. Such conditions must be promptly diagonsed and treated. Accuracy of judgement and reflex are most important for auto drivers, to avoid accidents.

(f) To ensure ideal standard of personal hygiene, to detect cases of skin diseases, patch pigmentation, depigmentation and anaesthesia of leprosy, sign of venereal diseases, unexplained weight loss, etc. Persons are advised and guided for further needful in such cases.

(g) The recording of hospitalisation with diagnosis, duration of stay, major pathological finding, accident, major injùry, deformity, etc. to the medical history sheet, so that the documentation helps in granting service and financial benefits to the policeman.

(h) Record of immunisation and other protective and prophylactic measures taken. Record of communicable disease already suffered in past, childhood is also important.

The above enumeration is neither complete nor total. The medical examiner may use his own clinical acumen to help the troops in maintaining disease free high standard of health. Practically, all the systems must be assessed by bedside methods and exert maximum effort to discover any pathological or serious ageing process during the annual medical examinations.

Verbal caution is sufficient for minor health problems, bad habits, addictions where as all major points must be recorded in appropriate columns. The medical officer may discuss with the Company Commander regarding health problems of troops and other hygiene and sanitation matters before submitting the report to the Unit Commandant.

The follow up action on the report of annual inspection of troops is a co-ordinated action by the Unit Commandant, Coy Commander and the Medical Officer. The persons detected with notable defects are disposed up in one of the following ways :

(a) Minor ailments or personal hygiene, cleanliness, etc. are verbally advised to person concerned on the spot.

(b) Persons with treatable conditions are advised to attend sick parade and report in hospital or M.I. Room for further observation, investigation and treatment as per requirement. Deserving cases are admitted to hospital for regularity of treatment. Communicable conditions are isolated from lines.

(c) Conditions for which the investigation or treatment facilities are not available in the unit level, such cases are referred to bigger hospitals of own force or nearby civil/military hospital for complete cure of his ailments.

(d) The chronically ill cases are listed and periodically reviewed. They can be allowed to perform duty with regular treatment with minor excuses for limited period. Cases who cannot bear the rigors of duty in field area or such sustained duty which may cause serious deterioration of his health may be recommended for posting to static institution, peace area or rehabilitated with proper duty in the unit.

(e) Cases suffering from permanent deformity, incurable disease, incapacitating illness and those who have no hope of returning to full duty even after prolonged treatment are produced before the Medical Board. The board shall be conducted as early as possible after administrative approval so that the fate of the person is decided to avoid loss of man-days, to give him benefits of service and sickness and to suitably fill up the post.

(f) Some of the invalidated cases are found suitable for jobs of less laborious nature. They are re-employed in non-government or regimental institution like welfare centres, montessory school, vegetable garden, gas agency, temporary stall man-in sports events etc. depending upon his degree of incapacity.

The system is good enough to monitor the health of fighting troops and to expose presence of any disease process, nutritional deficiencies, effects of age on various systems, mental state, abnormal behaviour, etc. in men when the exercise of medical inspection is performed meticulously. But due to various factors, the work is never complete nor is it done with enough professional sincerity. Once the defects are detected the men are not given sufficient scope to get their defects rectified.

Men away on leave, duty, sports are bereft of this facility. Some persons literally escape the departmental health scrutiny as they are out of unit for months together on sports duty. There is always a group who bypass or avoid to pass through the annual screening in fear of losing the job on detection of disease. Some hide their sexual or venereal diseases in fear of punishment.

Though, it is a co-ordinated action of Unit Commandant, Coy Commander and the Medical Officer, the work is left to the Medical Officer's responsibility who has no direct administrative control over the troops. It will not be out of place to say that this most vital health/survey exercise of the force should not be treated so lightly as a routine official formality and a well co-ordinated action of all the sections of the force will go a long way in maintaining the health and fitness of hard-working troops.

3. Medical Inspection of Food Handlers

In armed police forces, the food is served from a common kitchen, to men staying single in barracks. Whenever food is prepared on a large scale, the handlers are many and chance of contamination is more. The persons engaged in kitchen service such as cooks, water man, mess *sipahis*, mess under officers are potential source of large number of diseases. They act as carriers for parasitic diseases like round worm, tape worm, hook worm, amoebiasis, infective hepatitis, entric fevers (Typhoid & para-Typhoids), Gastro-enteritis, cholera, bacillary dysentry, infective diarrhoea, food poisoning, etc. The water borne diseases further adds to the list. Diseases like poliomyelitis, iodine deficiency, arsenic and lead poisoning, flurosis, etc. are through contaminated water. Any food handler suffering from such diseases is a potential danger to the community he is serving. Some of them are not sufferers but carriers, and they are also equally dangerous.

The periodic inspection of these food handlers of police force, kitchen includes detail physical examination of each individual to identify evidence of any external or internal disease, state of their personal hygiene, knowledge of cleanliness, dressing of finger nails, trimming of hair, healthy skin etc. Besides examination (microscopic) of stool for evidence of intestinal parasites and blood for estimating haemoglobine standard are done every quarterly. The specific test to determine carries state of diseases like typhoid fever are carried out annually. In some centres the periodical administration of deworning drugs to these persons are taken up to ensure eradication of intestinal works.

The system is one of the best public health measure followed in the police forces. It is carried out meticulously in all Central Police organisation hospitals. The system is of more practical utility in field formations like duty battalions, detached companies jungle camps, sports meet, ceremonial parade contingent, congregations, etc. But unfortunately, the facilities for such tests do not exist in field areas. The cooks and water-carriers are the bussiest persons. They work from early hours of the day till late in the evening. They have no holidays. The work-load may increase anytime with influx of troops or recruits. They have practically, no time to get their *bona-fide* ailments treated nor can they bring their ailing families to the M.I. Rooms. The strict health measures would reduce the morbidity rate in the force substantially specially in respect of communicable diseases.

In fact, the procedure should not be restricted to food handlers only. There are a few other groups of employees, mostly group 'D' category, commonly termed as "followers", as also the potential source of infection of various types. They are the barbers, shoe-makers, *safai karmachari*, washer-man etc. All such followers and assisting staff should be brought under the fold of periodic health check-up. The large group of hospital staff (Group C&D) of police force hospitals handle all category patients and are prone to exposure to diseases like tuberculosis, infective and viral hepatitis and AIDS etc., due to handling of infected materials, clothings and linens. This category of workers should also be protected against possible diseases, in the greater interest of the police force.

4. Health Reporting of Officers

The Senior Officers of the forces are expected to be more educated, elite and health conscious. They supervise, manage and command the troops. They look into discipline, moral, operational efficiency and welfare over and above the administration, budgeting and training of the men in uniform. The nature of their job demands less of physical and more of mental exercise. Only health officers can give better leadership to the force. In course of their normal duties, they receive ample dose of stress and strain leading to development of disease processes. These disease processes when detected early can be managed better and the person can be saved from serious damage or catastrophic episodes.

With this concept in mind the Indian Army has long back started compulsory health check-up of all commissioned officers and the CPO's have started similar practice in seventies and eighties. Some state police, especially, their armed wings have also followed the footsteps. The system was already applicable to the All India Service Officers, as the annual confidential report proforma contains columns like "State of Health". The reporting officers do not dare to comment on the state of health without taking opinion of the medical officer, and when the required specialists and facilities are available, the report becomes more elaborate. The Medical Officer takes up complete clinical exmination of the Officer, test of acuity of vision, ECG, X-Ray of chest, routine examination of stool, urine and blood, bio-chemical tests of blood for sugar, cholestrol urea, etc. The doctor may direct for any other special test depending upon the clinical reports. The summary of the entire battery of tests is sent to the reporting officer under "Confidential" cover. The doctor also expresses his opinion in general terms like "Unfit for straneous duties", "needs better care and treatment", etc. The result of the whole exercise can of course be verbally told to the officer with reassurance, explanation of each adverse findings and precaution so that the treatment part is not neglected.

As a general observation, the order of the annual health assessment programme is not taken in the right spirit by the affected officers. They try to avoid to undergo these procedures unless they are compelled to do so. Apparently, the reason may be apprehension of adverse effect on the service career. Such officers forget the positive side of the system. Here the senior police officers fail to be "exemplary" for the troops under their command unless they themselves come forward for annual check-up. The effect of present day stress and strain to officers is not unknown to anyone. The incidence of coronary heart diseases, acid-peptic diseases, diabetes, hyper-tension, mental breakdown, cerebro-vascular stroke, etc. are very common in groups of Executives. The age has its own impact on the systems even in absence of diseases. Early detection of these and other conditions helps more satisfactorily in management. Whenever possible, ultras-sonography, stress test and echo-cardiography should also be included in the list of tests.

The system has many happy returns despite all misunderstandings. Judicious interpretation of medical opinion at all levels are expected with best interest of the force and the individual officer

5. Endurance and Quarantine Tests

On several occasions, the armed police force doctors are asked to forward their opinion on non-medico-legal purposes on the state of health or fitness of persons. All such purposes can be divided into two major groups, such as Endurance and Quarantine.

The test of endurance is done when the person is detailed to undergo training courses, participate in sports activities, moving for duties in high altitude, etc. In all such cases the individual is required not only to be in a disease free state but a reasonable degree of stamina, exercise tolerance and the potentiality to bear the hazards of extra strain and extreme climatic conditions are also required. The general medical examination is supplemented by visual, auditory assessment or any other special test the medical officer may feel to undertake as per the type of special training or exercise the man is to undergo. In extra streneous exercises like mountaineering, rock climbing, commando, un-armed combat, counter insurgency and jungle warfare courses, or participation of major sports events of National, International standard, it is important to assess both physical and mental state of the candidate.

The medical examination for the quarantine purpose is to avoid incoming of infection to armed forces camp by the influx of people from various sources. As a matter of principle, the new comers should not be allowed to stay in the barracks before they are declared fit but such strict control is usually not practicable for obvious reasons. The categories of persons who should be examined are :

(a) All men newly posted to the unit.

(b) Men returning from course, leave or temporary duty for the period of over a month.

(c) Men returning from leave on medical grounds.

(d) Troops returning from over-seas service, specially endemic areas of malaria, yellow fever, AIDS, under International Health Regulations.

(e) Troops and employees seeking extension in service beyond the age of super-annuation.

(f) Troops returning to barracks after undergoing imprisonment, POW.

(g) Civilians being employed in canteen, dairy farm, butchery, barber shop.

(h) Troops who have known exposure to infective environment such as hospital attendant, after home visit, in endemic areas.

(i) School children residing in camp soon after vacations or excursions, etc.

In practice, the above tests are frequently insisted upon but opinions not strictly adhered to. There is no ready test for stamina and endurance. In an on-the-spot clinical examination, the doctor can only ensure an apparent disease free state for any course or sports. Due to shortage of eligible candidates, even medically unfit candidates detailed at times, making the entire exercise meaningless. The medical branch is often pressurised to over look minor points and some opinions are obtained for their administrative convenience. So far as quarantine tests are concerned, strict control is hardly possible when the units are hard pressed for men to put on duty.

6. Hygiene and Sanitation Round

The inhabitants of police force camps including family lines and the institutions have the justified expectations from the station authorities to provide an ideal situation on matters of sanitation, environment, water supply, disposal of garbages, barrack maintenance, street lighting and other basic civic facilities. The authorities also try to keep all the aspects in spic and span condition. In army, the cantonment board which acts as the civic body looks after the general sanitations including the seasonal measures like anti-mosquito measures, stray dog control and a host of other subjects. The technical advice is given by doctors incorporated in the body. In every army cantonment, the Station Health Officer (SHO) is the technical authority to aid and advise the administrative and civic authorities on matters of public health. But in para-military camps, district police centres and the police training colleges, such organisations do not exist. Usually, the Senior Medical Officer of the Station Hospital is in-charge of hygiene and sanitation of the camp. The periodic inspections of different areas of the camp are organised with close collaboration of the medical and executive branches of all units located in the Station. Surprise checks are also conducted on receipt of complaints and reports are sent to the suitable authorities. The action on the report is taken by the concerned institutions. A monthly or quarterly co-ordination meeting is called by the Station Commander (Senior Most Officer of the Station) and all such points are discussed and as and when necessary, instructions, bulletins are issued. In case of epidemics, notification are issued with information to local, district and municipal authorities.

The above procedures and systems are the broad principles followed in almost every police forces. The sole aim of maintaining any procedure or tradition in the forces is to maintain uniformity, discipline and systematism in working pattern, and finally to maintain the ideal health standard of troops. Police forces are the dependable arms of Government in matters of law and order and public peace. Depending upon the nature of duties and activities, every force has their own systems and arrangements for disease free healthful living of their members. Every system has its own limitations. It is also recognised that every system or procedure adopted in any organisation at any point of time has to undergo modification and metamorphic changes, in course of time. All traditions are created with a purpose. All purposes finally merge in national purposes. Hence, *"Forces Live & Survive with Traditions"*.

10

Impact of Diseases on Police Duty

An earlier chapter has been devoted in the discussion of mechanism of development of occupational diseases in policemen, although the nature of police duty alone is not the disease producing factor. The policeman's life style, separation from family, nutritional value of food, tension from local anti-social elements and politicians, domestic and socio-economic factors have been the major contributors in the process. For a sick policeman, the hospital is the only respite. Inspite of prompt and effective treatment, the disease leaves permanent or residual effect on the suffering policeman in the form of weakness or incapacity, which has direct impact on the efficiency and proficiency with which he was performing his duty. When the same condition prevails among a larger group of policemen, the police efficiency is slashed down and it fails to control the local crime or law and order situation on its agenda. Since police contributes its muscular power to help the administration for its smooth running the stability of the government or administration is at stake. Hence, ultimately it is the effective police force which helps in good governance. For a police force to be effective, it needs to be healthy both physically and mentally.

The variety and pattern of sickness in the police forces are no different from the general public but has its own peculiarities and scar of occupational brunt. Every ailment they suffer causes damage to the general health, limitation in activities, loss of interest and aptitude in the duties, even after clinical recovery. Some of the common ailments are discussed in the following paragraphs classified under the traditional medical systems with their impact on duties.

Mental Health

Mental health comprises of social, emotional and intellectual well-being of the individual. A healthy, matured and integrated personality is the final product of healthy genetic endowments, healthy intra-uterine and extra-uterine development and comfortable socio-psychological environment to grow and learn. The incidence of psychiatric disorders in armed forces is most prevalent in young combats who lose their mental stability on entering the world of crime, civil operations, transborder operation, etc. It basically is the problem of adoptation and adjustment for some. But in others, it is the dose of stress they receive that decides the state of mind.

The cases of mental sickness in police forces, generally are present either in acute forms like hysteria, anxiety state, confusion, psycho-somatic disorders, manic depression, schizophrenia or in chronic forms like depression, paranoid escape, etc. A group of them may be 'malingering' mental illness which is encountered frequently in police forces. The conditions may lead to absentism, disobedience, abnormal behaviour, mishandling of arms and weapons, confabulation, over-talkativeness or hyperactive personality change. They cause potential danger to other members and finally the effect of their presence in the force environment is injurious to the psyche of other inmates. Identification of cases, treatment and final disposal should be taken up without delay. It can be prevented by proper selection screening, man-management, training and moral building. The presence of warning signal of mental breakdown in any armed police personnel debars him from handling any sharp instrument, fire arms and his activities are always to be watched to prevent suicidal or homicidal attempts. Abnormal behaviour and mental sickness are noticed more commonly in women wings in police forces as such lives are entirely new for the young recruits.

Cardio-Vascular Disorders

The population of police forces is formed of age group 18 years to 55 years or 58 years. They are enrolled after thorough medical screening and put to initial tough training programme. When the policeman is filtered through such scrutiny, large number of childhood cardio-vascular diseases mostly of congenital and some of the rheumatic group are eliminated. Hence, the cardio-vascular problems are mostly of hypertensive, athtoscslerotic and ischarmic actiology, the chief causative factor available to them is stress. The natural history of these ailments commensurate with the situation, life style, food and habits like smoking and alcoholism in the armed personnel.

The coronary heart disease and hyper-tension both share common epidemiological factors like age (40-60 yrs), sex (predominantly in males), modern industrialised and commercial society, efficient and conscientious professions (legal, medical, executive), mode of life (sedentry habits), obesity and high cholestrol diet, etc. Other risk factors are diabetes, kindney diseases, thyroid disease, etc. The preventive measures are not so effective because of diversity of factors. Hence, spotting of cases and their treatment and rehabilitation have been the mainstay of action by the physicians of forces as they cannot practically change nature of the duty or life-style. Men of forces with regular check-up can be warned of their vulnerability to diseases and the measures required can be explained. Adequate prevention reduces incidence and early detection prolongs life-span. In any cardiac disease, the limitation to physical activities causes loss of man-days, involves long standing drug treatment and finally surgery at an advanced cardio-thoracic centre. Regular check-up can bring out diseases in their silent and asymptomatic phase.

Policemen with these ailments are not fully prepared to face the challenge of the criminal society and disturbed law and order. Active policemen are rehabilitated by transfer to inactive cadres like clerical, supervisory or watch and ward duties. Change in life style, weigh treduction, smoking proper diet and regular check-up and treatment of associated diseases are part of both preventive and in-service management.

Respiratory Disorders

In the police forces, respiratory diseases of both allergic and infective nature are prevalent almost in all ranks and files. Infective conditions like chronic bronchitis, tuberculosis and allergic conditions like bronchial asthma are the few common problems worth mentioning.

The long years of barrack life, frequent change of climate, accommodation in tents in extreme climatic conditions and close to soil and dust, exposure to industrial climate, jungle climate are some of the salient causative factors of respiratory diseases in the active duty policemen. Acute bronchitis is the most common seasonal short term respiratory infective disorder in all the police forces which has the high incidence but low morbidity or man-day loss. But pulmonary tuberculosis requires long treatment, hospitalization, heavy loss of man-days and may lead to finally rehabilitation, invalidation or death. The effective modern drug therapy, prompt treatment and isolation of positive cases have substantially reduced the incidence in forces, changing the earlier pattern. Improvement of diet quality helps in improving the prognosis and early return to duty as even after clinical cure the patients of pulmonary tuberculosis fail to perform full duties because of harmful effect of anti-tubercular drugs, general weakness and poor nutritional supplement. Cost of treatment is also a heavy financial burden on the policeman. Most tubercular cases receive the initial dose of exposure from their family members or relations and spread in the barracks when they are full blown cases. Hence, immediate isolation from barracks, full treatment, dietary supplement, etc. are to be meticulously planned.

The allergic group of respiratory diseases have the most common manifestation as bronchial asthma. The cases are chronically ill with attacks of dyspnoic episodes called "Status" in winter or in cold climates. They get admitted to hospital frequently and survive with drugs, and on oxygen. Some cases show remarkable improvement in change of station. Now, tests are available to know the allergen and if such allergen is avoidable, that is the best form of treatment. If the vaccine for the allergen is available, the cases get radical improvement. But in all cases of bronchial asthma, the exercise tolerance reduces drastically resulting in chronic absenteeism, frequent leave and other administrative problems. Loss of man-days is heavy.

In para-military forces, the patients can be given a chance to change his station with all good intention. But some forces do not have enough of scope to do so as their deployments are along the belt of International borders or industrial establishments where the men are exposed to pollution and other climatic hazards, as in BSF or in CISF. Cases of occupational asthma in men of CISF guarding the industrial establishments specially those of textile, cement, asbestos, jute and carpet industries are not uncommon. Other respiratory conditions like chronic obstructive air-way diseases and emphysematous type have relative prognosis as per severity.

Neurological Disorders

Out of all neurological symptoms, pain is the most common one in all sections of public. Any degree of pain, irrespective of its anatomical site and pathology of origin, is a disturbing factor for members of police force on duty as the man has to be attended by the first available medical man at the earliest and a reliever has to be arranged for the period he is taken away for treatment. Even local pain, like dental pain or migraine can cause disturbance in the duty schedule. Every case of pain requires thorough case study before instituting systematic treatment.

Police personnel with epileptic fits prove dangerous as they may get convulsion any time. They cannot be allowed to handle fire arms, electrical equipment, sharp cutting weapons and cannot be allowed to go near water or fire. If the patient happens to be a driver, he cannot be allowed to drive a vehicle. If the fits are severe and frequent, the patient has to be admitted to a hospital and treated fully. The drugs of choice for epilepsy are mostly tranquilisers. The effect of such drug also prevents a person to perform police duty. Naturally, a policeman on regular anti-epileptic cannot be considered suitable for the job.

Thromboembolic cerebro-vascular accident occurs in patients with severe untreated hypertension leads to paralysis of limbs, speech defect, bowel bladder decontrol etc. When the damage is permanent and no chance of recovery is expected the person has to be considered for terminal disposal by the Medical Board. Tic and tremor are also disturbing neurological symptoms of some systemic pathological process, which interferes in the police duty. Treatable causes should be searched for full remedy.

Gastro-Intestinal Disorders

Active police duty is affected by quite a large number of gastro-intestinal problems. Due to frequent change of places, the standard of potability of drinking water and use of cooking medium in the common kitchen in police barracks are the common causes of this disorders. Conditions like acute gastro-enteritis, irritable bowel syndrome, ulcerative colitis, amoebiasis and other intestinal parasitic diseases are intermittently symptomatic. Anorectal conditions like piles, fistulla, fissure, etc. are sufficient causes to dissuade the policemen to use proper uniform and maintain smart turnout and posture, cycling or motor-cycling. Chronic blood loss deteriorates the general health of the person and finally leads to chronic illness. Temporary camps with tentage accommodation do not have proper hygiene and sanitation, as they remain close to soil and in extreme climatic cor tions, the police personnel suffer from this problem in large mber giving a picture of an epidemic. Such incidents are demoralising to the troops.

The system is susceptible to stress. The stress disorders of G.I. system chiefly includes acid-peptic diseases. Other factors which contribute heavily in such disease forming process are irregular good timing, the condiment rich food, cold slopy rice rich food, high starch-low protein food, alcohol, smoking etc. The people who are over-conscious, compulsive, perfectionist, tense, competitive and ambitious, suffer most from the syndrome. Periodic pain with hyper-acidity comes 2/3 hours after food. Frequent small meals and strict dietary regimen are prescribed for these patients which they can hardly follow. The untreated or half-treated cases show worse complication like ulceration, bleeding or perforation when surgery is the only answer. The symptoms greatly hamper police duty.

Orthopaedic and Joint Problems

The police forces are basically an exercising community struggling to keep themselves, fit throughout their service career. The story is similar with the sportsmen. But the joints have to undergo changes with advance of age, limiting their flexibility. Diseases like rheumatoid arthritis, gout, spondyletic changes of cervical, vertebral column, calcification of tendons, calcaneal spur and malunion of old fracture site, etc. cause painful movement of joints with habitual exercise and strainful duties. Pain, swelling and deformities lead to abnormal gait, posture and damages the smartness of policeman, besides affecting his efficiency in police duty. Association of acute rheumatic activities make him chronically sick and finally he has to abandon service.

The orthopaedic surgeons of police forces spend much of their time in treating unexplained chronic backache. There is no specific test to substantiate and pin point the causative factor but yet the patient remains symptomatic and tries to avoid work. Loss of man-days on this account is heavy. Hence, the patients of 'backache' in police forces post a real problem to the doctors and the force commanders.

Metabolic and Endocrinal Disorders

Nutritional deficiencies dominate the scene of diseases in this group. Multiple vitamin deficiencies, mineral and trace element deficiency are caused by several factors like common preparation of food for large number of policemen in barracks, non-availability of choice food to each individual and when various regional recipe are not included in the menu. The situation is visible more clearly in Central Forces deployed in far-flung hill bound places where eatables and dry-ration items are air-dropped. The tinned, canned and preserved food stuff lack in nutritional value and man suffer from deficiency diseases on a mass scale. A capsule containing multiple vitamins, minerals and trace elements are supplied to men for supplementing the demand. Trace elements like Iodine, Zinc, Chromium, Cobalt, Manganese, Fluorine are normally obtained from food and drinks and have a definite physiological role to play in the metabolism of the body. Deficiencies bring weakness, lassitude, anaemia with cardiac and skin problems hampering police duty.

The metabolic disease worth mentioning relevant to the police life is Diabetes. As a general belief, the exercising public of police forces are not expected to develop such disease, but it is observed since the last few decades that more and more cases of full blown diabetes patients are detected. The reason for such an odd observation is apparently because of more of detection facilities available now to expose the obscure cases.

Diabetics do show symptoms, including some serious ones like hypoglycemia which severely affects their normal police duty. But in the modern medicines like oral hypoglycemic agent or purified human insulin once a day shot, the diabetics are living full life and performing duties like their healthy counter-parts. Regular, check-up, diet control, regulated dose of exercise, drugs and change in life style have radially changed the outlook of patients. The cases of thyro-toxicoscio have most disturbing symptoms like palpitation, nervousness, weakness, weight loss, tremor and heat sensitivity, etc. Patients become restless and severe cases cannot perform duty. Such cases need regular therapy and intermittent check-up with thyroid function tests.

Skin Problems

The importance of skin lesions in police forces is much more than that in civil life, for many reasons. Firstly, the chronic skin diseases are nearly serious and harbour in man's person for years together. Hence, the treatment is also neglected, specially, when it is in covered part. Secondly, the duration of treatment is longer and rate of improvement is judged by the patient himself since it is visible. He does not take prolonged treatment thinking that the remedy is ineffective or the disease is not trouble-some. Thirdly, the policeman lives in a common barrack where the chance of spreading a contagious skin disease to his fellow inmates is much more through man to men contact, or indirect contact through clothings, soaps, combs, razor, cosmetics etc. And finally, because of the nature of job, the police man fails to contact his doctor at regualr interval and follow the hard regimen of drug therapy.

Chronic skin conditions like furunculosis, impetigo, sycoses barbas, tiniasis, fungal infection, scabies, contract dermatitis, nail and foot infections cause enough trouble to interfere in police duty. Acute conditions like synthetic socks-allergy, rifle oil allergy and adverse drug reactions (ADR) are seen, frequently, which affects duty and waste man-days. Death or invalidation due to skin problem is rare except when it may be advanced case of leprosy. But chronicity and incurability haunts both the physician and patient. Situations can be improved with high grade of personal hygiene, health education, case finding and full treatment. Men at high altitude should be specially careful to prevent chill bain, foot problems on long wearing of snow-boot, gum-boot, jungle shoe or even ammunition boots.

Contagious skin diseases are transmitted in police forces through the uniform articles when the used ones are issued again to the new comers. This has been reduced drastically when some police forces have decided not to take back any used uniform. Thorough inspection of skin including private parts during the annual health review should be done meticulously. Skin problems are still more disturbing to the sportsman than the other police personnels. On the basis of skin problems itself many outstanding sportsmen suffer in reduced performance record and finally retire from the world of sports.

Gynaecological Problems

The problems have been much elaborately described in other chapters in connection with police women and the sportsmen. Their marital status decides much of the gravity of problems. All the married policewomen are faced with the problems of proper child bearing and child rearing. The normal menstrual cycles are not sufficient cause to abstain from work. Clerical or home-guard grade ladies can easily opt out of work where as arm force combatants cannot do so. With advance of age, cystocele, rectocele, urinary incontinence, uterine prolapse etc. are seen. Menopausal disorders come late in the reproductive life. Among all catogeries of policewomen, problems like vaginal discharges, and moniliases candidiasis, are common. The unmarried girls of police forces have shown higher incidence of anxiety, neurosis hyper-tension and unwed pregnancies where as their married counterparts have more number of miscarriages, complicated pregnancies and surgical deliveries. In such situations long hospitalisation is required with loss of man-days.

The doctors engaged in the care of women wings of armed forces and other women troops are required to be dynamic to give them effective counselling on the matters of family planning, avoiding unwanted pregnancies, pre-natal and post-natal care and genetic counselling to reduce the incidence of gynaecological morbidity among them. Early diagnosis helps to decide a course of treatment and prevents complication.

Eye-Ear-Nose-Throat Problems (E.N.T.)

Police men require good eye sight for general purpose to shoot as well as to drive. Hence, vision should be adequate in all respect like near, distant and colour vision. Clerical grade require good near vision to perform scriptory work and auto-drivers require perfect colour vision to be efficient driver than their "general duty" counterpart who require good acuity and nightvision. Eye defects of policemen render them completely handicapped hence, a thorough screening by specialist is required, particularly, of the auto-drivers who have to follow the traffic signals day and night. Follower staff may manage with inferior visual standard except the painters who require ability to recognise pigmentary colours. Staff engaged in wireless communication and computer operations require sharp night and colour vision.

A good hearing power is also a good asset to the drivers as well as general duty policeman as such defects may lead to operational and traffice hazards. Any case of nerve deafness or irrepairable tympanic membrane rupture may lead to removal from active police duty and rehabilitation in jobs of lower category. Seasonal throat infections are common but the impact on duty is minimal. Permanent hearing loss is a common occupational hazard among the professional shooters.

Dental Problems

The common dental problem among policemen is dental pain. Its severity may vary with the degree of disease and actual pathology but cops may take excuse from duty on the pretext. Besides, immediate treatment of pain and the underlying disease, regular dental check-up is required to prevent uncalled for trouble. Periodic dental check-up concept is held in some troops. Dental carries, naturally falling-out of teeth, and girgivitis are some of the common ailments for which the policemen seek dental service.

Genito-Urinary Problems

The common urinary problems in the police patients are renal or urinary stones, chronic urethrities and all the venereal discases. The reno-vesicular calculus are often painful and make patients bedridden. The frequent change of location, use of water from unfittered source and scanty water intake lead to such stone formation. The concentration of urine gives rise to burning sensation in urinary passage effecting the duty schedule. Most venereal diseases go painless unless the neural structures are affected. Hence, they get neglected and patients hide the disease in fear of punishment. But they are potential carrier of the disease affecting their family members and future generations. Health education and case finding is the only answer to the problem. Identified cases can be treated with full causes of therapy for the patient and his or her spouse.

The association of venereal group of diseases such as syphilis, gonorhoea, chancroid, lymphogranuloma inguinale, lymphogranuloma venereum, venerial wrethritis, genital wart and balano-prosthtis in the armed forces are morally and ethically regarded as self-inflicted. The incidence of V.D. in a police force unit points directly of its bad discipline, low morale and lack of man-management. It is a major factor to determine the operational efficiency of troops. Lack of facilities for healthy recreation, bad company, ignorance of sexually transmitted diseases and their complications. Drag the men of police forces to the immoral path of visiting brothels. Separation from families for long time, boredom and monetary affordability attribute heavily for such high incidence.

Genito-urinary problems have not only visible impact on the duty of policeman, it brings ill reputation for the whole unit and its Commanders. The public image is tarnished and operational efficiency deteriorates.

A I D S

Aquired immuno-deficiency syndrome or AIDS, is relatively new found clinical entity in the medical world, now known to be caused by HIV virus, transmitted through sexual contact, receiving infected blood transfusion, and using infected syringe. The discase may also be transmitted from an infected mother to her unborn child. There are two important features of the disease which affect human subjects most. Firstly, its long chronicity with deteriorating condition in every system of the body creating favourable condition for other infective diseases to flourish. Secondly, the high communicability, multiplying the victims in a very short time. The initial few years of the disease remain silent and are not detected. Laboratory testing facility is not available so commonly. Contact of AIDS in police forces ruins the general health standard of the force, spreads easily through sex contact and infected syringes in hospital. Since there is no known cure to this disease, prevention is the only way out.

Malaria and Other Fevers

Malaria fever is known in India since centuries and its effect in community and armed forces has been devastating. The military history of the world speaks of down-fall of some mightiest empires by spread of malarial fever in their army. The rapid spread through female anopheles mosquito, the high incidence of morbidity and deaths ruins the potency, capability and efficacy of troops. The anti-malarial, anti-mosquito campaign in military and para-military police barracks have been undertaken at a war footing which has greatly reduced incidence. The NMEP has been a success story at the national level but it did not last long. Since last decade, the disease has taken reverse trend with less effectivity to anti-mosquito measures and classical anti-malarial drugs. Now no area of the country is spared. But the improvement in drainage system, relieve of water logging and other hygiene and sanitation measures in police camps has been found effective to control the mosquito population. Assam-Burma Zone was the most malarious region in the world.

Police forces fall easy prey to the malarial fevers because of nomadic life, unsuitable accommodation, no facility to fix up mosquito net, and long hours of guard duty. The casualties from malaria out-number that of enemy action casualties. Long morbidity, complications, poor prognosis, weakness, blood-loss etc. lead to heavy loss of man-days.

Other fever producing infections like typhoid, typhus, paratyphoid etc. require immediate medical attention, long treatment, hospitalisation and convalescent, rest period cause long absence from duty for the policemen.

Obesity

It is the excess deposit of fat in the body increasing the body weight more than 10% of the expected depending on the age, sex, height and stock. Initially, the extra-fat is deposited over the fat depots such as abdominal wall, buttock, thighs, etc. Further deposition extends to interstitial tissues in the body, bone marrow, around the heart, liver, spleen, kidneys and higher circulating blood lipids. Obesity is associated with various serious health hazards. They are easy victims of diabetes, gall bladder diseases, and ischaenic heart disease. Obesity decreases exercise tolerance and reduces smartness with ill fitting uniform in police forces. Dietary restrictions especially fat and carbohydrate reduction in calorific supply and exercise are the well known ways to overcome obesity. But once obesity sets in, it hardly goes totally with any measure but can be maintained with shaping of figures. Active police duty is greatly affected with unmanageable obesity. Cases of rapid weight gain may be due to systemic pathology which needs investigation and treatment. Scientific studies have proved that obesity is directly linked with life span. (Life line is inversely proportional to belt-line) The exercising police personnel when adopt sedentary duty, gain weight. Hence, regular exercise should be ensured.

Smoking

Heavy smoking, in any form like *bidi*, cigar, *hukka* or cigarette is harmful habit with addicting effect and produces diseases like lung cancer, emphysema, ischaemic heart disease, peptic ulcers, gastric-cacinoma, tobbaco amblyopia and tremour, etc. Its vaspo-spasm effect gives rise to thrombotic tendencies, sluggish hemodynamics, chronic bronchitis and finally on stopping it, the withdrawal symptoms occur. Poisonous substances like nicotine-carbon-monoxide and complex mixture of benzopyrim phenol, aldehydes, formic acid and benzoic acid are inhaled in the smoke of cigars. Many of them are carcinogenic which has convulsive affect on central nervous system, reducing efficiency for intelligent work, reduces longevity damaging red blood cells, leads improper growth and premature death of foetus in smoking pregnant women. These stressful effects of smoking should be explained in simple language to all troops to save them from the hazards.

Policemen, particularly, troops deployed in hilly and snow-bound areas do not get good quality of cigars and are satisfied with local tobacco preparations with greater addictive and harmful effects. Troops at high altitude suffer from frost bite and ischaemic limb syndrome. The conditions get worse in the smoking habits. Men are more susceptible to chronic pulmonary infections like TB and health standard of the troops goes down.

Alcoholism

The prevalence of alcoholism is wide-spread in police forces. Its value is controversial in respect of food or energy supplement but being used as a psychological "stimulant" in moderate doses in the troops over the ages. It produces initial sense of well-being and "will to do more", in troops employed in adverse conditions. Troops in high altitude and in winter, officially, receive 60 ml of Rum yeilding around 400 calories when the daily need goes as high as 5000 calories. On the other hand, if consumed in excess it produces harmful effect on organs, particularly, liver, heart and brain. Confirmed alcoholics lose appetite and substitute alcohol for food and hence, suffer from avitaminosis, alcoholic gastritis, liver necrosis and fatty degeneration. Regular consumption leads to dipsomania, delerium tremens, psychosis and walleian degeneration by demyelirating the nerve fibres. Effects like error of judgement, impulsive action, instability in decision-making is seen which damages the primary image of police forces. Besides, the morale and discipline of troops are ruined. It is punishable offence to be under the influence of alcohol when the police officer is on duty.

De-addiction schedule with coffee or cocoa in lieu of alcohol beverage must be started with nutritional supplement, motivation and health education young recruits must be imparted proper knowledge in their basic training.

The readers may find a change in lucidity of analytical style in this chapter as compared to the earlier ones. Also there is over-crowding of medico technical terms in these preceding paragraphs. The stand must be clarified. Firstly, the topics have their own vastness and specificity. The long and elaborate topics have been condensed to be expressed in minimum possible words. Hence, the use of specific terms without explanation were unavoidable.

Secondly, an attempt has been made to cover all the major systems although one had to skip over a large number of clinical entities with proven impact on the life style of the men in uniform, to cut short the length of the chapter. During revision of this chapters, our well-wishers have advised to prepare a separate volume on the theme of this chapter.

11

Odds and Ends

The police health care service is a composite profession. The security and health professionals have to play complementary and supplementary role to make the system work. "Health is a battle winning factor"-- a well established truth. The concept of police health care is much above the classical hospital practice of medical knowledge. It is the complex problem of total health delivery system covering all aspects of health like preventive, curative, promotive, restorative angles of individual and community at all stages from life to old early age, at all spheres a home, school, campus covering all three components of health-physical, mental and social well-being.

Much has been said in preceding chapters on the health keeping of policemen. In a welfare state where the policy of the government is aimed to provide medical care to the communities at State's cost, the society also expects its savior police forces to be equally healthy or possess sound physique. Questions are often asked as to whether the present medical set-up is prepared enough to meet the challenging needs of the ever growing police forces in the challenging law and order situation. The managers of the system must be abreast of the development of modern technology, pharmaceuticals, concepts of treatments and newer research findings in medicine, hospital management, and public health measures. Some working methods and concepts are discussed in the following paragraph. The police hospitals all over the country may think of implementing some of these suggestions for the benefits of all sections.

Specialised Hospital Management

The hospital management is now a well developed branch of study in which both doctors as well as non-medical graduates take training. This covers a wide range of subjects like sanitation, disinfection, procurement of hospital store, disposal of hospital waste, water supply, electricity, supply medical gas supply, health transport, hospital diet, heating and cooling arrangements, air conditioning, and renovation. Because of its diversity, the matter should be left to professional managers and the qualified doctors may be spared to concentrate on their clinical work than anything else. The police hospitals are small in size and full time management staff may not be possible to be posted. In that case, one qualified manager may be posted in a group of hospitals. Who periodically attends to the management problems and solves them through the junior staff. Each hospital must have a management board in which both medical managerial, maintenance and public service staff are members. The Periodic review meeting would help them solve the day to day difficulties and also planning, development, extension, budgeting, etc. Such arrangement would considerably relieve the burdens of medical scientists who may devote on clinical, teaching and research work.

Public Relation

The medical world is an altogether different world which the general public fail to evaluate, the hospital tries to provide the best possible service to its beneficiaries inspite of financial administrative or technical constraints. But such bottle-necks are not realised by the users of the hospital. Hence a shadow of misunderstanding develops due to communication gap. As the outcome of the process, the easiest thing the public can do is to defame the hospital, highlight its short comings and failures without realising their limitations. The press and media help them in wide publicity and any amount of classification never clarifies their delusion. The situation can be avoided by establishing a sound public relation cell which keeps in touch with public management, press, government departments etc. and continuously on the job of meeting the press, redressing public grievances, issuing bulletins, announcements through media, and to display advertisements on facilities, plans and programmes of the hospital. Any death in hospital is not due to negligence of doctors or hospital staff as the agrieved party describes it. Inspite of the most ideal situations, some cases of adverse drug reactions (ADR) do occur. Such incidents are part of routine hospital life for which none can be blamed. The role of public relation cell is quite vital in this respect.

Continuing Education

As already discussed, medical science changes very fast. The trend of changes has to be kept in track by every practicing doctor. It is only possible through continuing education. A common feature which is observed among the staff is that after acquiring basic qualification and joining a job, the doctors and hospital staff develop slackness and lethargy in their learning process. The general plea is lack of time and the cumbersome way of going through old text books. It is not a healthy sign. A regular refreshing and updating of knowledge is required in day to day practice. The following suggestions are made to overcome this problem.

(a) Subscription to useful professional journals, to cater the needs of doctors, specialists, para-medical staff and managerial staff. The journals can be circulated among staff.

(b) Attending seminars and symposiums in nearby institutions, where eminent experts of various field deliver lecture and hold discussion.

(c) Arranging clinical meetings in the hospital on a theoretical topic of usefulness or a case presentation followed by discussion.

(d) Exchange of professional experience with eminent medical educational or practitioner of the city by inviting him in regimental functions.

(e) Arranging film-show, video-show on medical topics in hospital periodically. Educational video cassettes are available on hire on various topics. Besides the multinational pharmaceutical companies circulate and arrange show on the usefulness of their products and various latest developments.

(f) Publication of periodical journals, news-letters, etc. covering various clinical events and their management, case reports, etc.

The isolated police hospitals in the remote localities and battalion M.I. rooms in field areas may get affiliated to the nearby group hospital, base hospital or civil hospitals to avail similar facilities as such arrangement may not be possible at their level. It will help them in self improvements, brushing of their knowledge and preparation for pre-PG admission tests or overseas programmes on foreign assignments.

Exchange Programme

When a hospital plans to establish a new specialised service department or start any advance treatment/investigations and the doctors and staff are not sufficiently trained or experienced in the new type of job, some doctors and staff are deputed to undergo the specialised training. For that purpose a reputed hospital inside or outside the country is contracted to train the personnel for a reasonable period. In addition to that, any of their specialist or trained staff are invited to work for some time in new hospital to guide the work. All these things are done through the Exchange Programme. Such programme help in development of new specialists, laboratory research programme, special operations and procedures. Police hospital should take advantage of such programmes for the benefit of their patients.

Collaboration and Adoptation

Smaller hospitals desirous of improving their services in various disciplines may enter into technical collaborations with renowned hospital or a bio-medical engineering manufacturing company who help them setting of equipment, staff training to handle them, maintenance and repair, etc. Besides the hospitals may seek adoptation by a local advance hospital or medical college hospital and receive guidance is day to day working in clinical and research work. By this the doctors of police force hospitals can get exposed to modern technology and advancement in various disciplines and participate in research work. Such arrangements are good for mutual benefits of both hospitals doctors and finally the patients at large.

Visiting Specialists

In the police force hospitals, the posts of doctors are limited and hence the scope of posting specialists also remain limited. Receiving patients occasionally, who may require specialist service also cannot be ruled out or prevented. Because of the diversity of specialities, it is not possible to engage all type of specialist of full time basis. Hence, a system of visiting specialist for a fixed number of visits every week or month should be arranged, to get regular services in the police force hospitals. When government hospital specialists are not available private consultants may be engaged.

Documentation and Data Processing

The Performance and efficiency of a hospital are assessed from the data and documentations. The hospital documentation includes records of clinical, diagnostic and therapeutic informations of every individual patients who attend the hospital. The data is categorised system wise speciality-wise, and disease-wise and preserved in the hospital record room, even after completion of treatment transfer of patient to other hospital or death and post mortem. Such documents are, periodically, compiled to prepare hospital data and reports are sent to suitable offices engaged in the demographic study, planning and research.

In busy hospitals the task is enormous and the staff for the job is limited. Unfortunately, much less importance is attached to the aspects of health records on which the future health planning depends. To overcome such difficulties, computers are engaged for documentation data processing and data preservation and help in making health statistics section run efficiently.

Alternate System of Medicine

The allopathy system of medicine is called the "Modern Medicine" and the other systems like Ayurveda, Unani Homeopathy, etc. are called the alternate systems. Needless to say that the nomenclature is misnomer as the so called alternate systems are also not less modern in their approach in patient care and therapeutics. They have also equally shared the responsibility of helping the suffering humanity. The Systems are equally effective and popular in the society. Hence, the systems cannot be outrightly overlooked as "not-modern". Now, all over the world, the systems are marching shoulder to shoulder with modern medicine.

Strangely enough, although all the systems of medicine treat the same human beings, for the same ailments their concept and interpretation of diseases, drugs, methods of management are altogether different. The systems do not have any common agreable point. Hence, to create treatment facilities by alternate system, the doctor, para-medical staff and drugs, etc. have to be arranged in the same hospital in a parallel wing. Although, the takers, may be few, the chronically ill-patients who are not much benefited by allopathy, sensitive to allopathy drugs or terminally ill patients on minimal care may try the systems. The benefit drawn in such manner will be in the greater interest of the suffering humanity.

Integrated Command and Control

As discussed earlier the medical services to the state and central police forces are provided from different sources. Even in the central forces, the different forces under Ministry of

Home Affairs who historically have link with the Central Government Health Services (CGHS) are now operating as independent bodies under their own organisations. Although, these forces have many things in common, there is no co-ordination or common programme planning, etc. on administrative and technical levels. Though complete unification of cadres and services may not be feasible and may affect the interests adversely, unitary command by common medical directorate, for control of para-military forces may help to improve the prospect in many ways. The disparity in service condition, uniformity in the services of hospital staff and establishing common CPO hospitals can be looked into. Such a directorate may work as the apex body for liaison with the Ministry of Home Affairs, Ministry of Health, Indian Medical Council, Indian Medical Association, National Pharmacy and Nursing Councils, World Health Organisation, UNICEF, Indian Council of Medical Research and all such allied organisations for various purposes of improving health care system, research, statistics, planning, inter-national collaboration like AIDS control, etc. Such a direcorate can issue common bulletins and news letters on health and related matters. It can co-ordinate epidemic control, environmental studies and be a real asset to the police organisation. Small police organisations like States, Railways and Non-uniformed police, dog squad, camel squad, etc. may seek technical consultancy from such organisations.

Modernisation

Every system undergoes wear and tear with passage of time and needs periodic modernisation. In other words, it is the process to do away with the old useless things which have outlived their utility, and to embrace new and more useful ones. Modernisation can be most relevant to any hospital as the medical science is ever changing. The scope of modernisation therefore, in any hospital is unlimited. It can be on diagnostic procedures, methods of patient care, ways of medicaments, equipments, furniture, documentations, operating room sterilization technics, library and so on. A hospital may really lose its lusture and may fail to serve to the fullest extent without modernisation. The beneficiaries are to develop confidence and faith in the hospital for its better image. This is most vital in cases of police force hospitals as the perfect hospital service keeps the morale of policemen in high profile.

Group Health Insurance

During service period the police force members and their families, dependants like old parents, dependant brother or sisters are treated by their departmental hospitals for free. But since the number of hospitals are few, the men are deployed in the length and breadth of the country, families are left at home towns, the facilities are availed only by a small section the vast population. It is felt that there should be some system or scheme through which more and more police personnel and their families can benefit, even after retirement, resignation or voluntary quiting of service or when stationed any where. To an extent of imagination the private and semi-government agencies like medic-aim, health insurance companies can come to their rescue. All members of police forces and their family members can be insured under such scheme at nominal premium and get the benefits as and when they require. Costly treatment, hospital charges, operation charges etc. can be covered under such schemes which goes beyond the affordable limit of the police man.

The Arm Chair Police Force

All of us are familiar with the journalistic usage of "arm chair politician" honourably describing the senior citizens of the society who have taken retirement from active public life and have been engaged in giving valuable consultation in the light of their experience and knowledge. Such advices and guidance are found to be invaluable for the people engaged in the active practice of the same profession. Similar "*Guru-sisya Parampara*" is inseparable from professions like medicine, law journalism, business, astrology and so on. The services of senior bureaucrats, technocrats, police officers, army generals and veterans of this field are utilised after their retirement from active service in many fields. If such practice can be adopted for the police forces, the concept would not be entirely wrong. Special appointments of senior, retired or in service police officers to head committees and commissions, teams and missions. Connections and corporations are always done to utilize his expertise. The utilization of services of retired army and police personnel for watch and ward duties in international borders of Rajasthan, Punjab, Gujarat, West Bengal and other border states is already on cards with the government.

The superannuation age in the CPO's is either 55 or 58 years but in State Police Forces it is mostly 58 years. Besides, large number of members of police forces are relieved from active duties on voluntary retirement, medical invalidation, resignation, etc. There, trained police persons who form a part of the civilian public constitute quite a large number, although, the exact figures are not available. These people have sacrificed the most active and productive part of their lives for the cause of safety and security of the nation as loyal and sincere police soldiers. They have served the mother land at the expense of their personal, social and familial comforts. Such persons after retirement cannot be rejected to be totally useless and left in the cold, surviving with the handful of pension on the present days, of rising cost of living. What is most disheartening is these former loyal patriots suffer from various illnesses after retirement. They can hardly afford proper treatment unless they have a dutiful, sympathetic and affluent heir.

The requirements of medical standard and physical fitness in police forces is much higher than for the civilian posts. Hence, a person found unfit or sub-standard in a police force can be found useful in private and vocational jobs. The persons ousted from Central and State Police Forces put together constitute a vast army of "arm-chair police force" in which men trained in various trades, sports and games, tactics, are available. A former policeman who lost a limb in accident or operations, would not be able to be an efficient member of police force but he can be a good instructor with cretches or artificial leg in a tailoring class, or can be a good stenographer. A man with poor vision may not be efficient a driver or shooter but can be an efficient-printer or bakery man. The concerned ministries and forces should make comprehesive plans to club them to utilize their services in the society for constructive purposes.

As already proposed to Central Government, housing colonies can be established in border districts and other sensitive parts of the country, gradually spreading to every district for resettlement of ex-policemen, as they can be useful in a number of ways. Some of them are summarised below :

1. To spend life after retirement peacefully in house acquired through the co-operative scheme, enjoying good company, harbouring hobbies and habits.

2. To prepare boys and girls to build up body and physical efficiency to enter various police, para-military and armed forces with sufficient motivation to work for the country with full loyalty.

3. To run efficient civil defence service in border districts to prevent infiltration and trans-border crime.

4. Ex-policemen trained in various trades like tailoring, shoe making driving, motor like tailoring, motor mechanic, carpentry, etc. can run their work and teach workshops in their trade to train the educated unemployed young men and women to earn their lively hood. Poultry farms, dairy farms, bakery, etc. can also be started with efficient management by them.

5. Promotion of games and sports among school going boys and girls so that talented candidates can be fed to district or state pool.

6. To utilize their services in the role of home-guards or territorial army on the wake of local disturbance of law and order, natural calamities, fire, local mela, rallies, VIP visits and communal tension, etc.

On establishment of such ex-policemen colonies the planners have to extend some basic amenities to them such as schools, children parks, clubs, fire-fighting training centres.

The most important aspect of the government departments should look into is the health care facilities to these retired police personnels. The arrangement can be through expansion service from the nearby police hospitals or by establishing medical aid centres in these colonies. The cost of medical treatment is quite high now-a-days. These facilities would provide them a good relief in the fag end of their life where the medical requirement increases manifold. The men with long police career contact disease due to the nature of job and life style, already discussed in earlier chapters. Advancement in age brings many geriatric problems affecting almost all systems of the body and when untreated, lead to irreversible complications. A full health care starts with prevention and ends with rehabilitation. The running of such ex-policemen organisation would be the ideal form of rehabilitation and the most suitable gesture to senior citizens of police community. And this will give rise to a new world of the *"Arm-Chair Police Force"*

BIBLIOGRAPHY

1. Raghavan, R.K. — Indian Police-Problems, Planning and Perspectives, Madhavan Publications, New Delhi

2. Cohn Alvin, W. (Ed.) — The Future of Policing, Sage Publications, London

3. Sharma, P.D. — Police and Political Order in India, Research Publications, New Delhi

4. Gupta Giriraj, (Ed.) — The Social and Cultural Context of Medicine in India, Vikas Publishing House, New Delhi

5. Mishra, S.C. — State Police Organisation in India (A Review), Director General, CRPF

6. Saxena A.P. (Ed.) — Training in Government-Objectives and Opportunity, Indian Institute of Public Administration, New Delhi

7.	Pandey, P.K. and Gupta, L.C.	Outlines of Sports Medicine, Jaypee Brothers, New Delhi
8.	Berkow Robert (Ed.)	The Merck Manual of Diagnosis, Therapy Merck Sharp and Dohme Research Laboratories
9.	DG, AFMS	Manual of Health for Army (1968), Manager Publications
10.	Subramanyam, Dr. S.	How Should we Design Our Forces for 21st Century, *Punjab Kesari*, 12 December 1992
11.	Mathur, Dr. K.M.	Police In India-Problems and Perspectives, Gyan Publishing House, New Delhi
12.	Ghosh, S.K.	Politics of Violence, Ashish Publishing House, 1992
13.	Khanna, K.C.	Maintaining Public Peace-Abuse ofr :. Military Forces *Times of India* 15 August 1984.
14.	Sinha, B.M.	Police and Society *Hindustan Times*, 21 February 1984
15.	Nayar, Kuldip.	Police Turn into a Mob, *The Tribune*, March 1984

Index